THE SAFETY BLUEPRINT

NICHELLE LAUS

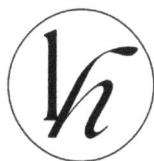

The Safety Blueprint
A Woman's Guide to Personal Safety and
Self-Defence From a Former Police Officer

Art Direction, including Typesetting and Layout Design Copyright © 2024 LeadHer Publishing.
Editing - Donna Zuniga

ISBN Print - 978-1-998411-17-7

To find out more about Nichelle Laus, visit nichellelaus.com

To find out more about LeadHer Publishing, visit leadherpublishing.com

lead*her*
PUBLISHING

DISCLAIMER

The information provided in this book is intended for educational and informational purposes only and does not constitute professional, legal, or personalized advice. While every effort has been made to ensure the accuracy and reliability of the content, the author and publisher make no guarantees or warranties, express or implied, regarding the outcome or effectiveness of the self-defence techniques and safety strategies discussed.

Readers are advised that personal safety and self-defence situations are unpredictable, and following the recommendations in this book does not guarantee the avoidance of harm or injury. Each person's circumstances and environments are unique, and individual results may vary. It is the reader's responsibility to

To all of you taking your personal safety into your own hands…
this book is for you.

INTRODUCTION

I HAVE WORN MANY HATS THROUGHOUT MY LIFE.

It has always been my passion and goal to help women bring out the best version of themselves through building confidence.

When I was a young girl, I was the victim of sexual assault for many years by a supposed trusted family member. After seven years, I finally found the strength and courage to become strong enough that no one could ever hurt me again. I started training and fighting in the amateur kickboxing and boxing circuit and continued my fighting, training, and coaching for over 25 years.

During that tumultuous period of trauma in my life, police officers were some of the very few people with whom I felt safe. I completely trusted them. This led me into my 15-year career as a police officer working general patrol, community services, working in high schools with high-risk students, in the criminal investigation bureau, public order unit, and more.

After resigning from policing, I dove into my passion of building confidence in others through health and fitness. Working with thousands of women, I watched every single one of them flourish and become the best version of themselves. I opened and co-owned a fitness facility in Toronto with my husband but unfortunately it became a casualty of the COVID-19 pandemic. The permanent closure of our gym space allowed me to return to my safety and self-defence roots. I opened up 416 Tactical Supply, an Emergency Services tactical supply store, and now share safety tips and self-defence techniques online for women who are looking for the confidence and strength to protect themselves on their own terms.

Throughout my journey I have also had the opportunity to navigate the ever-evolving landscape of media which allows me to connect on different levels with those who follow me. I have worked as a guest host, social commentator, fitness and safety expert, sponsored creator, and body double in traditional media and social media.

I have seen firsthand the unique challenges women face in maintaining their safety in today's world. From navigating public spaces to protecting our digital privacy, women often encounter risks that require us to be vigilant, informed, and prepared.

This book is a comprehensive guide to women's safety – drawing on my experiences, expertise, and the practical knowledge I've gained over the years.

Women's safety is not just about responding to immediate threats. It's about building awareness, confidence, and resilience. In the ten chapters that comprise the bulk of this book, we will explore a wide range of topics that address every aspect of safety – from situational awareness and self-defence techniques to cybersecurity, travel safety, and coping with trauma. Each chapter offers practical strategies, empowering insights, and real-world advice designed to help women take control of their personal safety.

As you read through this book, my goal is to arm you with the tools and knowledge you need to navigate life with greater confidence. Whether you're learning to trust your intuition, setting boundaries in uncomfortable situations, or developing a safety plan for solo travel, these strategies are designed to help you feel empowered and prepared.

Throughout your journey through this book, I want you to think of situations you have personally been in and how you navigated through each one. Ask yourself how you can take better proactive steps in your daily life to ensure your safety, and build the confidence to navigate challenging situations with resilience.

Together, we can create a safer world for women, one step at a time.

Stay safe,

Nichelle Laus

BONUS MATERIAL

Physical safety techniques are important to know, and explaining in written form is nowhere near as helpful as seeing these tools in action. I've created a complimentary video library as a bonus for readers of The Safety Blueprint.

Scan the QR code below, or visit **www.nichellelaus.com/bookfreebie** for videos and additional bonus materials that compliment the book!

BONUS VIDEO
TUTORIALS:

SCAN ME

CHAPTER 1

UNDERSTANDING PERSONAL SAFETY

WHAT *IS* PERSONAL SAFETY?

In today's world, understanding personal safety is more crucial than ever.

What is personal safety, anyway? Why should we, as women, have a keen interest in building awareness in this area? Personal safety encompasses a wide range of strategies, behaviours, and mindset shifts that are all aimed at reducing the likelihood of becoming a victim of crime or harm when in public environments.

Understanding personal safety requires that you incorporate different principles into your life so that you can empower yourself with confidence, resilience, and security in any situation.

Here are some principles that I think are important to consider when trying to understand personal safety:

Environmental Awareness

The first step in understanding personal safety is being aware of potential risks and threats in your environment. This includes recognizing common dangers such as street harassment, assault, robbery, and domestic violence. Understanding the factors that contribute to these risks − such as location, time of day, and situational factors − can help you make informed decisions to reduce them.

Intuition

One of our most powerful tools in personal safety is our own sense of "inner guidance" or "gut feeling" − which is our intuition. Especially as women who are raised to follow certain behaviours as we learn to function in society, we are often taught and conditioned to be polite and accommodating, even toward strangers. But in our ever-evolving society, it's essential to trust your instincts and prioritize your own safety above all else, even if it means being a little more blunt or assertive in your communication. If something feels off or makes you uncomfortable, don't ignore it. Trust your gut and take proactive measures to remove yourself from the situation.

Assertiveness

Assertiveness is another crucial skill for personal safety. Learning to assert yourself effectively can help deter potential threats and ensure your safety and overall well-being. Acting in a way that shows you are firm and assertive can help prevent potentially uncomfortable situations from starting or escalating because you are showing that you are not easily controllable. You should feel empowered to assert your boundaries firmly and confidently in any situation. This involves saying "no" when the answer is no, which sets clear boundaries with friends and acquaintances and helps support you in professional and social settings.

Situational Awareness

If you have ever heard me speak at an event or on one of my educational social media posts, you know two of my most commonly used words are "situational awareness." Situational awareness is the practice of being fully present and attentive to your surroundings at all times. This means paying attention to who is around you, where you are, and what is happening in your environment and settings. Avoid distractions that will compromise your ability to assess potential risks and respond effectively. Pay attention to what's going on in the environment that you're in, and try your best not to be oblivious to the situations and circumstances around you – especially when in public places where many people are around.

Safety Planning

Safety planning involves identifying potential risks and developing strategies to address them proactively (instead of reactively, which often leaves us stuck for any options if and when a safety breach is encountered). This may include planning safe routes when traveling alone, sharing your itinerary with a trusted friend or family member, and familiarizing yourself with emergency contacts and resources in your area. Having a safety plan in place can help you feel more prepared and confident in navigating various situations.

Self-Defence

While the overall goal of personal safety is to avoid dangerous situations whenever possible, it's also important to be prepared to defend yourself if necessary. Self-defence training can equip you with the physical and mental skills needed to protect yourself in the event of an attack. This may include learning basic striking and distraction techniques, as well as practicing assertive communication and de-escalation strategies.

Community

Finally, personal safety is not just about our own personal actions. It's also about building a supportive community that looks out for one another. You can enhance your safety by connecting with like-minded individuals, trusted friends, family members, neighbours, and community organizations. Having a strong support network can provide emotional support, practical assistance, and an additional layer of security in times of need.

COMMON MISCONCEPTIONS

Understanding personal safety does not come without misconceptions. These misconceptions can actually hinder your understanding of it. Some people feel that safety is strictly about physical protection. Although that is important, personal safety encompasses a broader range of factors including emotional well-being, mental health, financial security, and digital safety.

Another misconception of personal safety is that being cautious means you're paranoid or living in fear. In reality, being cautious actually means being aware of potential risks and taking reasonable steps to reduce them. Preparedness is key. One of my favourite sayings is: "It's about being *prepared*, not **paranoid**."

Some people think that dangerous situations only happen to other people, but everyone is susceptible to danger – regardless of age, gender, or background. Danger does not discriminate!

Another common misconception is avoiding certain places or people in order to guarantee safety. Although I do believe it is prudent to avoid high-risk areas or individuals when possible, danger can arise anywhere and at any time.

PERSONAL SAFETY – *FOR WOMEN*

As we continue to explore the topic of personal safety and the techniques and strategies required to build our toolbox of safety skills, we must recognize the unique position we're in as women navigating the often muddy and complicated waters of self-defence and personal protection. Learning about personal safety is different for women for a number of reasons.

Vulnerability to Gender-Based Violence

Women often face higher risks of gender-based violence – including harassment, assault, and domestic violence. An article from the Canadian Women's Foundation recently found that "even after controlling for other factors such as age and other individual characteristics and experiences, the odds of being victimized are 38% higher for women than men."[1] Understanding personal safety empowers women to recognize these risks and take proactive measures to mitigate them.

Unequal Power Dynamics

Societal norms and power imbalances often place women in situations where they may feel pressured to comply or feel unsafe asserting their boundaries. By understanding personal safety principles, women can assert themselves confidently and navigate such situations with resilience.

Empowerment and Agency

Knowledge of personal safety fosters a sense of empowerment and agency among women, enabling them to make informed decisions about their safety and well-being. This empowerment is essential for navigating both public and private spaces with confidence.

Breaking Stereotypes and Stigmas

Understanding personal safety challenges stereotypes and stigmas that place the burden of safety solely on women. It promotes a societal shift toward shared responsibility for creating safe environments, and challenging harmful attitudes and behaviours.

Self-Preservation

Personal safety education equips women with practical skills and strategies to protect themselves from harm. This includes recognizing warning signs, de-escalating tense situations, and knowing when and how to seek help or remove themselves from dangerous environments.

Creating Safer Communities

When women prioritize their personal safety, they contribute to the creation of safer communities for everyone. By being vigilant, speaking out against harassment, and supporting one another, women play a vital role in fostering environments where safety is valued and upheld.

———

Now, more than ever, it is important that we pay close attention to how we function in society and how we are prepared to protect ourselves should any danger arise in our surroundings. The prevalence of gender-based violence underscores the critical importance of prioritizing personal safety for women.

By fostering a culture of self-awareness, empowerment, preparedness (not paranoia!), and solidarity, we can navigate our environments with greater confidence and resilience, challenging harmful stereotypes and contributing to the creation of safer communities for all. Through education, advocacy, and support networks, women can assert their rights, dismantle systemic barriers, and cultivate environments where personal safety is upheld as a fundamental human right.

As we head deeper into the concept of personal safety in Chapter 2, we'll explore one of the most important skills conducive to a strong preparedness disposition: self-awareness.

---

1. Canadian Women's Foundation. "The Facts about Gender-Based Violence." Canadian Women's Foundation, 4 Jan. 2024, canadianwomen.org/the-facts/gender-based-violence/#:~:text=Women%20self%2Dreport%20violent%20victimization,higher%20for%20women%20than%20men. Accessed 7 May 2024.

CHAPTER 2

DEVELOPING SELF-AWARENESS AND CONFIDENCE

If you've never taken the time to learn about yourself intentionally, you may never have heard of the concept of "self-awareness." In this chapter, we will explore the critical role of self-awareness in enhancing personal safety, particularly for women. We will begin by defining self-awareness and examining how it contributes to situational awareness, enabling you to better recognize and respond to potentially dangerous situations. We will discuss how self-awareness helps build confidence and self-esteem, which are crucial for presenting a less vulnerable presence in public spaces. And, we will dig into the importance of cultivating intuition and assertiveness, which are essential traits for ensuring personal safety and empowerment.

NICHELLE LAUS

Learning more about who you are and what your personal strengths, traits, and tendencies are is a powerful tool for growing confidence and self-esteem, which can have a direct impact on how we behave and respond to potentially threatening situations.

WHAT *IS* SELF-AWARENESS?

Self-awareness is the conscious knowledge of one's own character, feelings, motives, and desires. It includes cultivating the ability to go inward and self-reflect on yourself and how your actions, thoughts, or emotions do or don't align with your internal standards. It's a deep understanding of the self in order to fully express your needs, desires, goals and preferences. It often involves recognizing one's strengths and weaknesses, emotions, thoughts, and how they align with one's values and beliefs. Self-awareness is the foundation of personal growth and is essential for developing a secure and confident sense of self. It allows individuals to understand how they are perceived by others and how their actions impact those around them.

Self-awareness can be divided into two types:

Internal Self-Awareness:

This involves understanding one's internal state, prefer-ences, resources, and intuition.

External Self-Awareness:

This involves understanding how others view us in terms of those same factors.

Both types are crucial for effective self-management and relationship-building. When individuals are highly self-aware, they can make informed decisions, respond to challenges with greater resilience, and navigate social situations more efficiently.

WHY IS SELF-AWARENESS IMPORTANT FOR PERSONAL SAFETY?

As discussed in Chapter 1, self-awareness plays a big role in helping us to cultivate a strong level of situational awareness. And, situational awareness is crucial for ensuring that we're observant and mindful of the people and environment around us.

The more self-aware we can be, the better equipped we are to understand if something in our surroundings feels off. This helps us to decide if we should take action to change our circumstances in order to prioritize our safety.

Being more self-aware is important as it not only helps us to recognize and avoid potential dangers or threats, but also helps us to improve our overall judgment (of situations and people), improve our sense of confidence and decision-making skills, and can even help us to recognize manipulative or questionable behaviour.

HOW TO BECOME MORE SELF-AWARE

Self-Reflection

Regular self-reflection is a powerful tool for increasing self-awareness. This can be achieved through journaling, meditation, or simply taking time each day to think about your actions, thoughts, and feelings. Asking questions like "*Why did I react that way?*" or "*What could I have done differently?*" can provide insights into your behaviours and underlying motivations.

Seeking Feedback

Constructive feedback from others can offer a different perspective on how one is perceived. Trusted friends, family members, or colleagues can provide valuable insights that might not be apparent from a self-reflective perspective alone. It's important to approach this feedback with an open mind and a willingness to learn.

Mindfulness Practice

Mindfulness involves paying full attention to the present moment without judgment. This practice can help you become more attuned to your thoughts and emotions as they occur, rather than being swept away by them. Techniques such as deep breathing, body scans, and mindful observation can enhance your awareness of your internal states.

Personality and Strength Assessments

Tools such as the Myers-Briggs Type Indicator (MBTI)[1], the Big Five personality traits[2], or the StrengthsFinder assessment[3] can provide structural insights into your personality traits, preferences, and strengths. These assessments can serve as a starting point for deeper self-exploration.

Energetic Assessments

There are many alternative wellness "energy assessment" modalities that you may consider exploring in order to better understand your unique energy "blueprint" and how you are designed to function in our society in alignment with your energetic makeup. These energy assessment tools typically leverage astrology and metaphysics to help explain how different people are well suited to different roles, hobbies, relationships, and more. Finding out more about your Human Design, your unique Gene Keys, or even exploring your astrology type may help you go deeper into building on your awareness of yourself and your personal characteristics.

Setting Personal Goals

Clearly defining what you want to achieve in various areas of life can clarify values and priorities. Regularly reviewing and reflecting on these goals can help you maintain alignment between actions and personal values, enhancing self-awareness over time.

SELF-AWARENESS TO ENHANCE SELF-CONFIDENCE

Self-awareness is a critical component in building and sustaining self-confidence. When you can understand your strengths and weaknesses, you can capitalize on your abilities and work on areas that need improvement, leading to a more confident and authentic self.

Understanding Strengths and Weaknesses

By being aware of your strengths, you can leverage these attributes in situations that call for confidence. For example, if you know that you are an effective communicator, you can confidently take on roles or tasks that require public speaking or negotiation.

On the contrary, recognizing your weaknesses allows you to address them constructively rather than being hindered by them. For instance, if you struggle with time management, acknowledging this issue can then prompt you to develop better organizational strategies, which in turn reduces stress and enhances overall confidence.

Popular author and business thought leader Marcus Buckingham has openly taught on the importance of focusing on your strengths and leveraging them so that your weaknesses can naturally lessen as you don't give them as much focus or priority. This is a great way to work on naturally incorporating more of what you're good at, so the things that you may not be great at can get less attention and thus, have less opportunity to expand or grow.

"Strengths-based thinking is a philosophy that might be summarized as follows:

- It's better to focus on building people's strengths than trying to fix their weaknesses.
- People can only perform at their best when they are in a role suited to their strengths.
- Strengths are those things we are good at and enjoy doing (not things we are good at but don't enjoy doing)." [4]

Focusing on your strengths can go a long way to enhance your self-confidence and self-esteem, and to continue building how well you know yourself as a human being – a.k.a, how self-aware you are overall.

Alignment with Values

Self-awareness helps you align your actions with your core values, leading to a more consistent and authentic life. When your actions are aligned with your values, you will feel a greater sense of integrity and self-respect, which boosts confidence. For example, if you value honesty and practice it in your professional life, you will feel more secure and self-assured because you know you are acting in accordance with your principles.

Emotional Regulation

A high level of self-awareness contributes to better emotional regulation. Understanding your emotional triggers and responses allows you to manage your reactions more effectively, reducing feelings of becoming overwhelmed and increasing resilience. This emotional stability, in turn, translates into greater confidence in handling various life situations.

Building confidence through self-awareness is extremely important as it relates to consciously improving your personal safety strategy. It may not seem like something that is directly related to safety, but a woman exuding confidence (on the surface) in a potentially dangerous interaction can help to minimize how much the situation escalates, versus a woman who comes off insecure and by default, more vulnerable.

The term "fake it 'til you make it" comes to mind here, and as much as I want you to build a solid foundation of *real* and *true* confidence in your life (not just for "show"), showing up in a more confident light – even if you don't yet *feel* truly confident – is a key personality characteristic that can help protect you in difficult situations. Self-confidence gives off a different energy than insecurity and can make a big difference in regard to how you appear in public and in society.

TRUSTING INTUITION AND GUT FEELINGS

Intuition, often described as a "gut feeling," is the ability to understand something instinctively, without the need for conscious reasoning. It's a form of immediate cognition that can provide critical insights for decision-making, especially in situations where quick judgment is necessary.

Understanding Intuition

Intuition is informed by past experiences, knowledge, and instinctive understanding. It's the subconscious mind drawing on a vast array of information to make quick – yet often accurate – judgments. For women, trusting their intuition can be particularly important in situations that pertain to personal safety and well-being. I always say: "Trust your gut, it never lies!"

HOW TO TRUST AND DEVELOP YOUR INTUITION

Developing and trusting your own "inner-guidance radar" (a.k.a, your intuition) can significantly enhance your decision-making process and overall sense of self-awareness. By learning to listen to your body, reflecting on past experiences, practicing mindfulness, keeping a journal, and taking small risks, you can work to fine-tune your intuitive abilities. Let's explore some of these strategies for developing a better sense of intuition.

Listen to Your Body

Physical sensations often accompany intuitive feelings. A knot or butterflies in your stomach, a quickening pulse, or a feeling of unease can all be indicators of your intuitive response to a situation. Paying attention to these signals can help you interpret what your intuition is trying to tell you.

Reflect on Past Experiences

Reviewing past decisions and their outcomes can provide insights into how intuition has guided you previously. Think about a time that you have had a gut feeling. Did you listen to it and were you correct? Understanding patterns in your intuitive responses can build trust in this inner guidance.

Mindfulness and Quieting the Mind

A busy mind can drown out intuitive insights. Practices such as meditation and mindfulness can help quiet the mental chatter, making it easier to hear and trust your intuition.

Journaling

Keeping a journal of your intuitive experiences and the decisions based on them can help reinforce the reliability of your gut feelings. Over time, you'll see how intuition has played a role in your life, which strengthens your confidence in it.

Take Small Risks

Start by trusting your intuition in low-stakes situations. As you see positive results, you'll build the confidence to rely on it in more significant circumstances.

ASSERTIVENESS/FIRMNESS

Assertiveness is the ability to express one's thoughts, feelings, and needs directly, openly, and honestly, while respecting the rights of others. It's a crucial skill for maintaining healthy relationships and protecting one's boundaries, which is essential for personal safety.

HOW TO DEVELOP ASSERTIVENESS

Know Your Rights

Understanding your personal rights is the first step to becoming assertive. This includes the right to express your opinions, to say no without guilt, and to ask for what you need.

Practice Saying No

Being able to say no is a fundamental aspect of assertiveness. Practice this by starting with small requests and gradually working up to more significant ones. Remember, saying no is about respecting your own boundaries.

Use "I" Statements

Communicate your feelings and needs using "I" statements. For example, "I feel uncomfortable when…" or "I need more time to decide." This approach reduces the likelihood of the other person feeling attacked.

Maintain Eye Contact

Good eye contact conveys confidence and sincerity. It helps ensure that your message is taken seriously.

Practice Assertive Body Language

Your body language should align with your words. Stand or sit straight, maintain a relaxed posture, and use gestures to emphasize your points.

Role-Playing

Practice assertiveness in a safe environment through role-playing. This can help you prepare for real-life situations by providing a rehearsal space where you can experiment with different responses.

———

Self-awareness and self-confidence are deeply intertwined, each enhancing the other in a positive feedback loop. By cultivating self-awareness, you will gain a deeper understanding of your strengths and areas for growth, align your actions with your values, and improve your emotional regulation.

For example, when I was in my early twenties, I worked as a computer programmer at an insurance company.

I often found myself in situations where I felt uncomfortable or uneasy but lacked the self-awareness and assertiveness to address them effectively. One particular incident stands out vividly and has become a cornerstone in my journey toward developing greater self-awareness and assertiveness.

I was the youngest on the team, eager to prove myself and keen to be seen as a team player. During a team meeting, my supervisor assigned me a project that I felt was well beyond my capacity, both in terms of time and skills. Instead of voicing my concerns, I nodded in agreement, not wanting to appear incapable or unwilling.

As the days and weeks went by, the pressure of the project began to take a toll on me. I was working long hours, sacrificing personal time and sleep, yet I was still unable to meet the unrealistic expectations. The stress was intense, but I kept pushing myself, not realizing how detrimental this was to my well-being and productivity.

One evening, after another exhausting day, I broke down in tears, overwhelmed by the mounting pressure. It was then that I realized I needed to change my approach. I started reading about self-awareness and assertiveness, seeking to understand why I had allowed myself to be placed in such a situation and how I could prevent it from happening again.

I began by reflecting on my actions and feelings. I kept a journal where I noted down instances where I felt stressed or uncomfortable, and I tried to identify the triggers and my responses. This practice helped me to recognize patterns in my behaviour and understand my limits better.

With growing self-awareness, I realized the importance of setting boundaries and communicating them effectively. Gradually, I started applying these skills at work.

A few months later, a similar situation came up. My supervisor once again assigned me a challenging project. This time, however, I calmly and confidently proposed a more realistic timeline and suggested additional resources that could help me to meet the project's demands and deliverables.

To my surprise, my supervisor was understanding and agreed to my suggestions. This experience was empowering and reaffirmed the importance of being assertive and self-aware.

Throughout my life and career as a police officer, the benefits of developing self-awareness and assertiveness have been profound. I became more confident in my abilities and more aware of my limitations.

I can communicate my needs and concerns more effectively, which has led to healthier work relationships and better job performance. I am no longer afraid to say no when necessary, ensuring that I maintain a balanced and healthy lifestyle.

Building self-awareness and assertiveness has transformed how I handle challenging situations. By understanding myself better and confidently voicing my boundaries, I have been able to navigate my professional and personal life more effectively. This journey has taught me that it is not only okay to speak up for oneself, but essential for long-term success and wellbeing.

---

1. Briggs Myers, Isabel, Mary H. McCaulley, Naomi L. Quenk, and Allen L. Hammer. *MBTI® Manual: A Guide to the Development and Use of the Myers-Briggs Type Indicator Instrument*. 3rd ed. Palo Alto, CA: Consulting Psychologists Press, 1998.
2. Wiggins, Jerry S., ed. *The Five-Factor Model of Personality: Theoretical Perspectives*. New York: Guilford Press, 1996.
3. Buckingham, Marcus, and Donald O. Clifton. *Now, Discover Your Strengths*. New York: Free Press, 2001.
4. "In a Nutshell: Strengths-Based Thinking." *Human Performance Technology by DTS*, 26 May 2014, blog.hptbydts.com/in-a-nutshell-strengths-based-thinking-strengths-movement. Accessed 27 May 2024.

CHAPTER 3

NAVIGATING PUBLIC SPACES SAFELY

Navigating public spaces safely is crucial for everyone, but especially if you're an identifying woman, you may face unique challenges and risks that others do not, simply by virtue of the stereotypical perception of vulnerability associated with womanhood. This is why, in Chapter 2, we discussed the importance of improving your overall self-awareness to build confidence, self-assuredness, and being more assertive – even if just *appearing* so to start, as it significantly reduces the opportunity for others to perceive you in this more vulnerable light.

Understanding situational awareness, implementing safe travel tips for both urban and rural areas, and employing effective nighttime safety strategies can significantly enhance personal security. This chapter explores these aspects in detail to better equip women with practical knowledge and actionable techniques for staying safe.

WHAT IS SITUATIONAL AWARENESS?

I touched on situational awareness a little in Chapter 1, but to refresh your familiarity with the concept, situational awareness is the ability to understand and interpret what's happening around you in real-time. It involves being aware of your surroundings, recognizing potential threats or changes, and understanding how these elements might affect your safety or goals. Essentially, it's about knowing what's going on so that you can make informed decisions and respond effectively. It's such an important principle when considering your personal safety. It involves being conscious of your surroundings and understanding what is happening around you. It allows you to identify potential threats and react appropriately, before situations escalate.

The great thing is that situational awareness is a skill that can be developed and made sharper with practice. Let's learn more about how we can do this effectively in order to become better at consciously managing our awareness of situations, circumstances, people, and events around us at all times, regardless of the setting.

KEY COMPONENTS OF SITUATIONAL AWARENESS

Developing situational awareness requires an understanding of its three key components: **perception**, **comprehension**, and **projection**. These components work together to provide a comprehensive framework for recognizing and responding to danger, allowing individuals to maintain control and make informed decisions in various environments. By mastering the elements of situational awareness, women in particular can enhance their ability to stay safe and confident in any setting.

I want to give you a few examples of how having poor situational awareness can be dangerous for you, especially if you're a woman who has never experienced any potentially threatening situations. The tendency is to think "That won't happen to me," or, "Things like that don't happen where I live," – but you would be surprised at what can happen if you aren't consciously making an effort to pay attention to your surroundings. This doesn't mean that you need to become paranoid, refuse to trust anyone, or look at your surroundings with fear; rather, it means that you should step up your level of observation and be aware of the things you can do to ensure that you aren't going to be caught off-guard in a dangerous situation. The more prepared you are, the more you can influence your own personal safety.

———

Case Study: Emily

Emily was walking home from work, completely absorbed in her phone, texting and scrolling through social media. She had her headphones on, was listening to music, and was totally oblivious to what was happening around her.

As she approached a busy intersection, she didn't notice that the "Don't Walk" sign was lit. She stepped off the curb just as a car came speeding around the corner. Thankfully, a passerby saw what was happening and shouted at her to stop.

Emily jumped back onto the sidewalk just in time, her heart racing. She realized then how close she had come to being seriously hurt, all because she wasn't paying attention to her surroundings.

Now, she always makes a point to put her phone away and stay alert, especially when she's walking through busy areas. It was a real wake-up call for her about the importance of situational awareness.

———

Case Study: Farah

Farah was leaving a late dinner with friends and walking to her car in the parking lot. It was pretty dark, and she was busy rummaging through her purse for her keys, not really paying attention to anything else.

Just as she was about to unlock her car, she heard someone call her name from a distance. It was another friend from dinner who had come out a bit later and saw what was happening.

Farah looked up, saw the person getting uncomfortably close, and quickly got into her car, locking the doors behind her. The person immediately turned and walked away, probably realizing that they had been spotted.

That close call made Farah realize how important it is to stay aware of what's happening around her, especially in less secure environments. Now, she always keeps her head up and her keys ready, making sure she knows who and what is around her before she gets to her car.

As you can see, situational awareness can have to do with the innocent dangers that don't involve anyone else but can become dangerous if you aren't paying close enough attention (like stepping out onto a street), as well as the dangers of potentially threatening people whom you do not know, who could have one of many ulterior motives that could involve you being physically, mentally, or emotionally hurt (like an unidentified person approaching you without consent).

When it comes to people and interacting with those you do not know, the purpose is not to make you untrustworthy or to think every stranger you come across has poor intentions; it's simply to ensure you know what to do if someone is exhibiting questionable behaviors or crossing personal boundaries, like approaching you when you're alone at night in an otherwise empty parking lot. A person who approaches in that situation could just be asking for directions or inquiring about where you just ate your dinner...but we can never be too careful and I would much rather you be a little skeptical than completely aloof. It is important that we work to find a happy medium and a healthy balance because it could save your life.

SITUATIONAL AWARENESS TECHNIQUES

Building upon the foundational understanding of situational awareness, it is essential to delve into the practical techniques that can enhance your ability to stay alert and safe in various environments.

Situational awareness techniques are specific strategies and behaviours that help you maintain a high level of vigilance, enabling you to detect and respond to potential threats effectively.

These techniques are designed to be integrated into daily routines, making them second nature and ensuring that safety remains a priority. By learning and practicing these techniques, women can significantly improve their ability to navigate public spaces with confidence, reducing the risk of becoming targets of crime.

Maintain a Baseline

Establish what is normal for your environment. Knowing the baseline helps you detect anomalies or unusual behaviour.

Scan Your Surroundings

Regularly scan your environment, especially in unfamiliar or crowded places. Use a 360-degree awareness technique by briefly checking behind you as well.

Trust Your Instincts

If something feels off, trust your gut. Instincts are often based on subconscious observations.

Stay Focused

Avoid distractions like excessive phone use. Stay alert and attentive, particularly in transit hubs, parking lots, and secluded areas, particularly if it is nighttime.

Observe Behaviour

Pay attention to the behaviour of people around you. Look for signs of nervousness, aggression, or anyone paying too much attention to you.

Plan Your Routes

Know your routes and exits. Familiarize yourself with the layout of places you visit frequently. Have an exit plan in mind whenever possible.

Use Reflective Surfaces

Use windows and mirrors to check your surroundings discreetly.

Leverage Technology

If you feel unsafe, use the technology you have to your advantage. If you're carrying your phone, call a friend or partner loudly, or open up the camera and start openly recording what's happening that is making you feel unsafe. These actions can deter potentially threatening people from pursuing their initial plans. *Note, please do not record people publicly without their consent unless you truly feel threatened or unsafe, for personal safety reasons ONLY.*

Keep a Safe Distance

Maintain personal space and be aware of anyone invading it.

Stay Prepared

Think about potential scenarios and have a plan. Know how to respond if something goes wrong.

SAFE TRAVEL TIPS FOR URBAN AND RURAL AREAS

Traveling safely requires an understanding of the unique challenges posed by different environments, whether bustling urban centres or calm rural landscapes. Urban areas often present risks related to high population density, traffic congestion, and potential crime, while rural areas may pose challenges due to isolation, limited services, and unpredictable terrain.

By implementing tailored safety strategies for both urban and rural settings, women can enhance their personal security and navigate these diverse environments with greater confidence.

This section offers practical travel tips designed to address the specific risks associated with each setting, providing valuable guidance for ensuring safe and secure journeys regardless of the destination.

STAYING SAFE: URBAN AREAS

Stay in Well-Lit Areas

Stick to well-lit, populated streets and avoid shortcuts through alleys or deserted areas.

Use Public Transport Safely

Wait in well-lit, busy areas and sit near the driver or in crowded sections. Avoid isolated train cars.

Stay Alert

Avoid wearing headphones or being engrossed in your phone. Be aware of your surroundings and people nearby.

Limit Distractions

Keep your valuables secure and avoid showing expensive items like jewelry or electronics.

Buddy System

Travel with a friend when possible, especially at night or in unfamiliar areas. Have a plan in place with this buddy for procedures you will both know and follow should a suspicious situation arise.

Know Emergency Contacts

Have local emergency numbers saved on your phone. In Canada, you can use 911 for emergencies.

Blend In

Try not to stand out. Dress appropriately for the area and avoid flashy accessories.

Avoid Sharing Personal Information

Be cautious about discussing personal details or travel plans in public.

Use Ride-Sharing Apps Wisely

Verify the driver's identity and share your trip details with a trusted contact.

Research Your Destination

When preparing to travel to an urban destination you have never been to, do your research in order to identify potentially unsafe areas or locations. We have amazing technology available to us now that makes looking into popular areas in advance readily available and accessible. Look up the address and neighbourhood/zone where you'll be staying, check social media apps for content creators who give location-specific tips and advice, and connect with local residents for more information on what to expect in your area.

Case Study: Courtney

A friend of mine recently shared a story with me about her experience of feeling unsafe in an urban centre, and I think it will help to expand on how pre-travel research, consulting with locals, and being self-aware and intuitive can mitigate unsafe situations. With her permission, here's what happened:

"In 2019, I traveled to San Diego, California to attend a popular women's business conference with a group of my friends and fellow female entrepreneurs. We pre-booked our six-person accommodations on a popular and trusted travel site and as directed, arrived at the general "zone" where we were told the house was located based on the booking. This "zone" was on the outskirts of the downtown area, and the address brought us directly in front of a small cafe.

As competent, tech-savvy people, we were stumped at where we were supposed to check-in to the property we booked. We were using the available technology, address, maps, and the app itself to try to connect with the homeowner to find the physical location. We didn't seem to be in the right place based on the address we were given, and we were dumbfounded. We'd all used this app with great success in the past, and could not understand what we were doing wrong.

*When we finally reached the host of the property, we were told to go to a completely different location that was not within walking distance and would require travel of over 10 kilometres further into the city; an **entirely** different location than what was disclosed originally.*

Upon hearing this, something felt off. We collectively felt that this last-minute adjustment to the location area was fishy. We agreed that it was odd to be asked to go to another "zone" completely and wondered why that was the case.

We were in a public place, it was daytime, and we were a group of six women – so we acted safely and with permission, asked two of the cafe employees and a few local latte-sipping customers for their thoughts on the new location we were told to go to.

*We received six consistent answers: **do not** go to that area, it is unsafe. Full stop.*

Every single person we asked for feedback echoed the same sentiment and feared that the original "zone" was not shared on the listing for fear of discouraging people (who know the area) from booking the property altogether.

As obvious tourists (each of us with a full suitcase in tow), we trusted that the local people – who had zero involvement in our trip and nothing to gain by misleading us – were being honest in their feedback. We took their cautions seriously and adjusted our next actions accordingly.

Immediately, we got on the phone with a company representative who agreed something was off and promised to find us comparable alternative accommodations so that we did not have to further compromise our safety and feelings of unease. As we were in the process of finding an alternative, the homeowner caught wind of our last-minute cancellation and was openly furious with our actions and ultimate decision. He sent several inappropriate messages trying to deter us from making the decision to change and tried to threaten us with reprimands, fees, and charges we would apparently be liable for should we go through with our new plan.

We continued to trust our collective intuition and confirmed with the company representative that we would not be penalized in any way by making this choice. We wound up at a lovely home in a quiet and more suburban area that not only felt safer, but gave us the peace of mind to enjoy our trip with confidence and avoid a potentially dangerous environment.

If we weren't willing to question the instructions we were given, to trust our gut instincts, and to follow up with the company regarding their policies and procedures before blindly obliging to this sketchy host's demands, we could have found ourselves in a very different situation with a potentially dangerous outcome.

Trust your gut; use the technology available to you; don't be afraid to double-check or ask about things you aren't aware of; and always take action and make decisions with confidence and assertiveness, even if you might make someone unhappy by virtue of your choices. You should never be made to feel like you don't have a choice or should blindly comply with someone else's demands, especially when you're in a place that you know little about."

———

STAYING SAFE: RURAL AREAS

Plan Ahead

Rural areas may have limited services and less frequent public transport. Plan your route and check schedules in advance.

Stay Connected

Ensure your phone is charged and consider carrying a portable charger. Cell service can be spotty in remote areas.

Tell Someone

Inform a friend or family member about your travel plans, route, and expected arrival time.

Know Local Services

Familiarize yourself with local emergency services, nearest towns, and safe places to stop.

Carry Essentials

Bring water, snacks, a flashlight, and a basic first-aid kit. These can be lifesavers in isolated areas.

Vehicle Safety

If driving, ensure your vehicle is in good condition and you have a full tank of gas. Carry a spare tire and emergency kit. If you live in a climate that has varied temperatures, be sure you have wool or emergency blankets packed in the car in case you are without heat.

Dress Appropriately

Wear weather-appropriate clothing and sturdy footwear.

NIGHTTIME SAFETY STRATEGIES

Navigating public spaces at night can present unique safety challenges, as reduced visibility and fewer people around can increase the risk of potential threats. For women, adopting specific nighttime safety strategies is crucial to ensure personal security and peace of mind.

This section explores a range of proactive strategies designed to enhance safety and provide a greater sense of control and protection during nighttime hours.

Stick to Busy Areas

Walk in well-lit, busy areas. Avoid deserted streets, parks, and shortcuts.

Walk Confidently

Walk with purpose and confidence. Keep your head up and make it clear that you are aware of your surroundings.

Stay Connected

Keep your phone easily accessible. Use apps to share your location with a trusted contact.

Use Personal Safety Devices

Carry a whistle or a personal alarm device. Know how to use them and keep them accessible.

Check-In Regularly

If you're walking or traveling at night, check in with a friend or family member at regular intervals.

Avoid Isolation

Stay in groups or public places. If you must wait for transport, do so in well-lit areas with other people around.

Know Your Route

Plan your route in advance. Avoid poorly lit areas and know where you can find help if needed.

Use Ride Services Wisely

Verify ride-sharing details, such as the driver's name and vehicle license plate. Sit in the back seat and lock the doors.

Be Cautious with Strangers

Be cautious when approached by strangers. Keep a safe distance and be firm if someone makes you uncomfortable.

Stay Sober

If you're out for the evening, limit alcohol consumption to stay alert and in control. If you've been drinking, arrange for a trusted friend to accompany you or use a reliable ride service. Never leave your drink unattended.

Trust Your Instincts

If you feel unsafe, act on your instincts. Find a safe place or seek help immediately.

Seek Safe Havens

Identify safe places along your route, such as 24-hour stores, police stations, or well-lit public areas where you can go if you feel threatened.

Avoid Distractions

Stay off your phone and avoid using headphones. Being alert increases your ability to detect and react to potential dangers.

Navigating public spaces at night requires heightened vigilance and proactive measures to ensure personal safety. As women, we can enhance our overall security by sticking to well-lit, busy areas, walking with confidence, and staying connected through phone apps that share our location.

PAUSE: PERSONAL SAFETY FOR KIDS

While this isn't a book about the safety of children specifically, I want to pause here to note that the things you're learning in this book are helpful for you, but are also key personal safety concepts that you can teach your children about, regardless of their age or gender orientation.

The sooner our children can learn about self-aware-ness, confidence, assertiveness, and situational awareness, the better equipped they will be to navigate potentially threatening situations and environments as they grow up.

For example, teaching your kids to practice heightened awareness when returning to your vehicle after shopping in a busy place, or to be vigilant about scanning their surroundings when walking down a busy street (in lieu of looking down at technology and being completely oblivious to the people and spaces nearby) are key initiatives that can have a major positive impact on how they grow up with personal safety in mind.

Being proactively safety-oriented can also help children feel more confident to take action should something threatening to their safety arise, like a stranger interacting with them in a store or at the playground.

For example, proactively setting up a code word should a stranger try to manipulate them into believing their parent(s) asked them to engage with them. Or, setting specific parameters and role-playing how they should respond if someone ever tried to influence them in some way in public (like loudly yelling "HELP! THIS IS NOT MY MOM! THIS IS NOT MY DAD!"). These actions can outright deter a person from taking their intentions any further because as soon as they think a child might know what they're up to, they're less likely to actively pursue their initial actions.

This is a great time to reflect on what you have learned so far, and share your acquired knowledge with your kids, family, friends, and female colleagues.

———

In the next chapter, we will begin to explore strategies for managing harassment in many different ways, so that you can take an active approach to your personal safety and reduce the potential for situations to escalate into more dangerous territory.

CHAPTER 4

DEALING WITH VERBAL HARASSMENT

On a typical Tuesday evening, Rachel decided to stop by her favourite café after work. She cherished these moments of solitude, enjoying a cup of coffee while reading her latest novel. The café was bustling with the usual after-work crowd, creating a lively yet cozy atmosphere.

As Rachel settled into her seat by the window, she noticed a group of men at a nearby table. They were loud and boisterous, clearly enjoying their evening. At first, Rachel paid them no mind, focusing instead on her book. But soon, she felt their eyes on her.

One of the men in the group began making comments loud enough for her to hear.

"Hey, sweetheart, why don't you smile more? You'd look so much prettier."

Rachel tried to ignore him, her heart pounding a little faster. She kept her eyes on her book, pretending not to hear. But the comments persisted, becoming more intrusive and uncomfortable. The other men started piping in, so now there were four of them shouting different comments in her direction.

"Come on, don't be shy!"

"How about you join us? We won't bite."

"You're looking good today, what gym do you go to?"

Rachel glanced around, hoping someone else in the café would intervene, but everyone seemed engrossed in their own conversations. The tone of the group started to grow more insistent and less friendly, cutting through her attempts to block them out.

*"What's **wrong** with you? You too good to talk to us? You think you're better than us?"*

Rachel felt a mix of fear and anger bubbling inside her. She wanted to stand up for herself, to tell him to back off, but she also worried about escalating the situation and what might happen if she spoke back to the group. She considered leaving, but the thought of walking past their table made her uneasy.

What should Rachel do?

Verbal harassment is a common issue that affects women in various public and private spaces. Understanding what verbal harassment entails, how to respond to catcalling and unwanted attention, setting boundaries assertively, and using verbal de-escalation skills are essential for maintaining personal safety and psychological well-being.

In this chapter, we'll explore these critical topics to empower you with the knowledge and tools needed to handle verbal harassment confidently and effectively.

WHAT *IS* VERBAL HARASSMENT?

Verbal harassment refers to unwanted, unsolicited, and often aggressive or demeaning comments, remarks, or gestures directed at an individual. It can occur in various settings, such as on the street, in the workplace, on public transport, online…or at your favourite local café, even when other people are around who you think might be supportive or helpful of the situation, but aren't. Verbal harassment can range from seemingly innocent comments to explicitly threatening or abusive language. It can escalate quickly and turn from "seemingly innocent" to "potentially dangerous and threatening" at the flick of a switch.

Verbal harassment has many impacts from emotional distress, to reduced confidence, and behavioural changes. Understanding the nature and impact of verbal harassment is the first step toward addressing and mitigating its effects.

TYPES OF VERBAL HARASSMENT

Catcalling: Unsolicited comments, whistles, or gestures typically made by strangers in public spaces.

Unwanted Comments: Remarks about appearance, attire, or personal life that are intrusive or offensive.

Sexual Remarks: Inappropriate comments about a person's body or sexual propositions.

Threatening Language: Verbal threats or aggressive statements intended to intimidate or coerce.

Insults and Name-Calling: Demeaning or derogatory language aimed at belittling or humiliating someone.

RESPONDING TO CATCALLING AND UNWANTED ATTENTION

Catcalling and unwanted attention are common forms of verbal harassment that many women experience in public spaces.

I have experienced this type of public harassment in the past, and I know just how unpleasant and scary verbal harassment can be. It makes me feel anxious, frustrated, and embarrassed. For some women, it can have profound and lasting effects on their emotional, psychological, and social well-being. The immediate feelings of fear, anger, and embarrassment can evolve into long-term consequences such as chronic stress, mental health issues, and changes in behaviour and life choices.

Recognizing these serious impacts is important for developing strategies to support women and to create safer environments.

Can you think of a time when you were verbally harassed? How did it make you feel? How did you respond? Did you feel like you were stuck, backed into a corner, or had no way out? Did you think bystanders would help you, but didn't? Did you feel your heart racing, or scramble to make a phone call or pretend to see someone you knew in order to protect your safety? Responding to these behaviours effectively requires a balance of assertiveness, situational awareness, and self-protection strategies.

When it comes to personal safety, the circumstances regarding your unique situation will make all the difference. Being verbally harassed in a public place is very different from being harassed somewhere where there is nobody else around. Being approached in daylight versus at night can also change the dynamics of your available options. I hope this section can provide you with some basic information to assist you in feeling more confident evading the harassment no matter what situation you're in. As always, these are broad suggestions and your plan of action will vary depending on your unique circumstances — but keep these strategies in mind and do your best to prepare and avoid potential situations where you could be left alone and are more susceptible to this kind of harassment.

Ignore the Harasser

Often, the safest and most effective immediate response is to ignore the cat caller and keep moving. This minimizes the attention they receive and can prevent escalation. Try to get somewhere that has more people around, if you're in an isolated place. Pick up your pace slightly if need be.

Stay Calm and Composed

Maintain a neutral facial expression and avoid showing anger or fear, which can sometimes provoke further harassment. If you don't appear to be afraid and come off as more unbothered than fearful, you're less likely to be an "easy mark" or target. Harassment like this works based on the power dynamic. If the harasser does not think they can have control over you by creating fear, they may back off.

Use Body Language

Non-verbal cues such as shaking your head, holding up a hand in a "stop" gesture, or giving a firm look can communicate that the behaviour is unwelcome.

Verbal Responses

If you do respond, aim to be as direct, firm, and brief as possible: Use clear, firm statements to assert your boundaries. For example, "Stop talking to me," or "Leave me alone." As much as you may feel like you'd like to lash out, refrain from using insults or aggressive language. That can just escalate the situation and bring more unwanted harassment.

Enlisting Bystander Support

While you won't always be able to use this technique, it's an important one to mention and a skill I teach women to utilize regularly whenever possible. Enlisting bystander support can be an effective strategy to reduce the threat of verbal harassment by leveraging the presence and support of others, even if they aren't aware of what's going on at the time. Here's how you might do this:

Make Eye Contact and/or Signal for Help

Look around and identify someone nearby who seems approachable. Make eye contact and use nonverbal cues like a wave or nod to signal that you need assistance. Sometimes, simply making someone aware of the situation can prompt them to step in.

Speak Up Clearly

If making eye contact isn't enough, address the bystander directly in a calm and clear voice. For example, say, "Excuse me, could you please help me? I'm feeling uncomfortable."

Use Assertive Language

Clearly state what you need from the bystander. For example, "Could you stand here with me for a moment?" or "Can you help me by calling the café manager over?"

Describe the Situation

Briefly explain what's happening so the bystander understands the context. For example, "This person has been making unwanted comments, and I'm feeling threatened. Could you stay nearby until they leave?"

Create a Safe Environment

If possible, move closer to the bystander or a group of people. Safety in numbers can deter the harasser and provide you with immediate support.

Thank the Bystander

Express gratitude for their assistance. This not only acknowledges their help but also reinforces the idea that stepping in was the right thing to do.

MITIGATING HARASSMENT OPPORTUNITIES

When it comes to the potential threat of any kind of harassment, it's a good idea to think in advance about the following things in general, so you're less likely to wind up in a space where you are alone and away from potential safety.

Plan your route to ensure it includes well-lit and busy streets, and use maps or navigation apps to find the safest paths. Choose parking spots close to entrances, in well-lit areas, and preferably in busy parking lots, avoiding isolated areas, especially at night. If possible, travel with a friend or colleague, especially in the evenings or when going to unfamiliar places, as there's safety in numbers. When using public transportation, wait in well-lit and populated areas, sit near the driver or in a car with more people, and move to another seat if you feel uncomfortable in any way – even if the "vibe" just feels "off." (That's your intuition!)

Walk in the middle of the sidewalk, away from doorways, alleys, and bushes where someone could be hiding, and avoid shortcuts through alleys, parks, or other isolated areas. Try to schedule your activities during daylight hours and, if you need to be out after dark, let someone know your plans and expected return time. Carry a small flashlight or use your smartphone's flashlight app to help you see better and make you more visible to others. Wear clothes and shoes that allow you to move freely and quickly if needed, and avoid items that could restrict your movement or attract unnecessary attention.

Keep your head up and be aware of your surroundings; avoid distractions like looking at your phone while walking; and trust your instincts – if something feels off, leave the area. Have a safety plan in place, including knowing where the nearest safe locations are and having emergency numbers readily accessible.

Consider using safety apps that can share your location with trusted contacts, alert authorities, or provide other safety features. If you're unfamiliar with an area, avoid exploring it alone, especially at night, and stick to places where you know there will be other people around.

I know this seems like a LOT of prep work and planning to avoid something that may never even happen to you, but it's better to be prepared for anything than to be oblivious to what could potentially escalate into a very serious situation.

PERSONAL BOUNDARIES

Setting boundaries assertively is crucial for managing verbal harassment and protecting your personal space. Assertiveness involves expressing your needs and rights clearly and respectfully without being passive or aggressive.

Setting boundaries and learning to be assertive can be challenging for many women due to societal conditioning, fear of conflict, and a desire to be liked or accepted. However, developing these skills is essential for personal well-being and safety. I suggest practicing assertive techniques in other areas in your life until you are comfortable with protecting your personal space and well-being. It can take some time before you feel comfortable enforcing your boundaries in an assertive way, but trust me — it's worth exploring for your overall safety in any situation.

Use "I" Statements

Frame your boundaries using "I" statements to take ownership of your feelings and avoid sounding accusatory. For example, "I don't like being spoken to that way," or "I feel uncomfortable with your comments."

Be Clear, Direct, and Calm

State your boundaries simply and directly, and speak in a calm tone to ensure your message is understood. For instance, "I want you to stop making comments about my appearance."

Maintain Eye Contact and Repeat If Necessary

When safe to do so, maintain eye contact to reinforce your message and convey confidence. If necessary, repeat your statement in the same calm manner.

If the situation escalates, prioritize your safety and look for exit routes or seek help. Take a mental note or record details of the harassment that can be useful if you decide to report it to authorities later.

DE-ESCALATION STRATEGIES

De-escalation refers to the process of reducing the intensity of a conflict or potentially volatile situation.

The goal is to calm the individuals involved, preventing the situation from escalating into violence or further hostility. De-escalation techniques aim to create a safer environment by using calm and controlled responses, thereby diffusing tension.

Verbal de-escalation, then, specifically involves using verbal communication strategies to defuse a potentially aggressive or hostile situation. This approach focuses on listening, calming, and redirecting the conversation to prevent an escalation. Verbal de-escalation techniques include maintaining a calm tone of voice, using open and non-threatening body language, validating the other person's feelings, and setting boundaries in a respectful manner.

During my policing career, verbal de-escalation was a technique I frequently used in situations. Verbal de-escalation techniques are essential because they reduce the intensity of a conflict or potentially violent situation, ultimately promoting safer outcomes for everyone involved.

Oftentimes, it's the tone in our voice and the non-threatening body language that can help diffuse a situation. Stay composed yet direct, and maintain a neutral posture without crossing your arms or clenching your fists while speaking. This, of course, is easier said than done, because often when emotions (and tensions) are **high**, emotional intelligence is **low**. It can be difficult to stay composed and remember your verbal de-escalation techniques when the stakes are high. This is why it's a good idea to practise these techniques and role-play them in advance so that you feel more comfortable and confident taking action if and when the opportunity arises.

———

Let's consider how Rachel might use some of the tips and strategies from this chapter to mitigate the potentially threatening situation she is in with the verbal harassment she is experiencing. She needs to de-escalate the situation and can use several techniques in order to do so.

As explained earlier, first Rachel tries ignoring the men's comments. In this case, her approach was unsuccessful. They kept bothering her.

If that's the case, next I'd suggest Rachel keep her composure, adjust her body language, and use firm, straightforward words and signals to ask the men to stop speaking to her because the comments are unwanted. Assuming the men do not listen to her requests and continue to disrespect her boundaries, I would suggest she consider what else she can do to remove herself from the situation safely.

She could either approach a cafe employee for support or look around the area to see if anyone else might be able to give her a "safety in numbers" advantage, effectively leaning on bystanders for support. If there is a person or group nearby that she can signal with eye contact or even approach the person or group unprompted, she can gain an advantage.

Rachel could head to a table of 2-3 people (or just 1 person if that's all that's available) and use clear, loud speech to explain that she is feeling uncomfortable. She could say something like:

"Excuse me, could you please help me? I'm feeling uncomfortable with the comments these men are making."

Or,

"Would you mind standing here with me for a moment? Your presence would really help."

Or,

"These men have been making unwanted comments, and I feel threatened."

The acknowledgement of another person, as well as publicly mentioning the unwanted behaviour in question, is likely to get the group of men to back off and retreat, realizing Rachel is no longer as fearful or vulnerable as they first thought.

As much as I wish this wasn't our reality, verbal harassment can happen anywhere, anytime – from busy cafes to parking lots, sidewalks, malls, supermarkets, and quiet parks. Your response strategies will need to adapt to the unique circumstances of each situation. Whether you're setting boundaries, using verbal de-escalation techniques, or enlisting bystander support, it's essential to be prepared. Practising these tips and strategies in advance can also help you to feel more confident and better equipped to handle harassment if and when it occurs.

Remember, the goal is to maintain your safety and peace of mind, ensuring that you can navigate public spaces with confidence and assurance. Stay aware, stay prepared, and always prioritize your well-being.

CHAPTER 5

SELF-DEFENCE TECHNIQUES FOR WOMEN

U p until this point, things haven't gotten physical. We are about to head into some strategies for self-defence and personal safety that are more physical in nature. We will explore self-defence techniques and the subtle differences in these techniques when employed specifically for use by women. We'll also discover basic physical defence methods, practical training exercises, and the legal implications of using self-defence.

By equipping ourselves with these skills and knowledge, we can better protect ourselves and feel more confident in our ability to navigate potentially dangerous situations.

SUBTLE DIFFERENCES IN TECHNIQUES FOR WOMEN

When it comes to self-defence, the techniques that women employ can differ subtly yet significantly from those commonly taught in general self-defence classes. These differences stem from the unique challenges and physical dynamics women often face in threatening situations. Understanding these distinctions is crucial for women to effectively protect themselves. Here are a few things to keep in mind as a broad overview of how techniques differ for women versus men:

Targeting Vulnerable Areas

Women should target vulnerable areas such as the eyes, nose, throat, and groin. These areas are sensitive and can distract an attacker regardless of their size or strength. Other techniques that involve manipulating small joints – like fingers – can be highly effective for women, as these do not require significant strength but can cause considerable pain and compliance.

Leveraging Body Mechanics

Women can use leverage and technique to overcome physical strength disparities. Techniques that involve using the attacker's force against them such as throws and joint locks are particularly useful.

Balance, Speed, and Agility

Maintaining a low centre of gravity can provide better stability and balance, making it harder for an attacker to overpower or knock down the defender. A flexible and balanced stance also allows for quick transitions between offence and defence, helping women to react swiftly to threats.

Women can use their agility and speed to their advantage, employing rapid strikes and evasive manoeuvres to create distance and disorient the attacker.

Psychological Tactics

Techniques that involve surprising the attacker, such as pretend compliance followed by a sudden counterattack, can provide a critical advantage when defending oneself. Using assertive verbal commands to set boundaries and de-escalation strategies like the ones mentioned in the previous chapter can also help in situations before they become physical.

BASIC PHYSICAL DEFENCE TECHNIQUES

Drawing from my 20 years of experience competing in boxing and kickboxing, I now regularly leverage the skills and strategies learned in these sports to teach women effective self-defence techniques and personal safety. The core principles of these combat sports – such as striking, movement, and defensive manoeuvres – are highly applicable to real-life self-defence scenarios.

My general approach to self-defence focuses on foundational moves that prioritize safety, leverage natural body mechanics, and capitalize on quick, decisive actions. By mastering these straightforward techniques, my students can build confidence and competence, empowering themselves to respond effectively in real-life situations without the need for complex or overly elaborate manoeuvres.

Here, I will provide an overview of some of the movements you can practise to be better prepared to protect yourself. However, it'll be hard for you to picture the exact movement I'm describing without seeing it visually.

To ensure you get a clear picture of how to move your body to master these techniques, I have created a free video companion series that includes demonstrations of each of the movements described in this section.

This comprehensive library of video tutorials will help you better understand how to leverage your body to protect your safety in various situations.

FREE BONUS MATERIAL

Scan the QR code below, or visit **www.nichellelaus.com/bookfreebie** for videos and additional bonus materials that compliment the book!

BONUS VIDEO LIBRARY

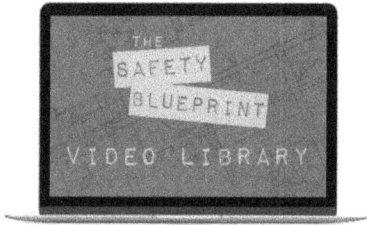

SCAN ME

STRIKES AND PUNCHES

In self-defence, understanding and effectively using different strikes and punches can be crucial for personal safety. Striking and punching in strategic ways help you to leverage various parts of the body to deliver forceful blows that can incapacitate an attacker or create an opportunity to escape. This section introduces some key techniques, and each of these movements utilizes the body's natural strengths and can be executed with minimal training, making them practical and powerful tools for self-defence.

Palm Heel Strike

Delivered with the heel of the palm to the attacker's nose or chin, causing disorientation and pain.

Knee Strike

A powerful upward strike with the knee aimed at the groin or midsection, which can incapacitate the attacker quickly.

Elbow Strike

A highly effective strike with the point of the elbow that can be thrown sideways, upwards, downwards, diagonally, or in direct movement.

Shin Kick

A straightforward kick to the attacker's shin designed to create distance and disable the attacker.

ESCAPES FROM GRABS

Knowing how to escape from various grabs can be vital for ensuring your safety. Grabs are common tactics used by attackers to restrain or control their victims, but with the right techniques, you can break free and protect yourself.

This section will cover methods to escape from common grabs, providing you with the skills to quickly and effectively respond to these threats. By mastering these escape techniques, you can increase your confidence and ability to stay safe in dangerous situations.

Wrist Grab Release

When someone grabs your wrist, the key is to break their grip using leverage, not strength.

Instead of pulling directly back, drive your elbow forward and rotate your arm towards the attacker's thumb, which is the weakest point of the hand.

Bear Hug Escape

If someone grabs you from behind in a bear hug, wrap your own arms over theirs and drop your weight down. This will make it harder for your attacker to lift you.

Distract them with a foot stomp or shin kick and a head butt. Lift a shoulder and rotate out the same side controlling their wrist to create enough distance to escape.

Front Choke

If someone grabs your throat from the front with both hands, it's important to act quickly. Take your hand, extend your first two fingers and drive it through the attacker's arms to their throat as hard as you can.

If you can't use your fingers, you can always use an open hand and strike them in the throat with the area between your index finger and thumb.

Headlock

If someone puts you in a headlock, avoid panicking and keep your airway clear by taking one of your hands and placing it on their wrist to release some pressure on your neck. With your other hand, pinch the attacker's inner thigh area as hard as you can, or strike their groin with an open hand upward chopping motion.

Simultaneously, twist your body towards them while stepping around them to loosen the hold. As you twist, slip your head out from under their arm, and follow up by moving away or countering with further strikes.

Mount

If you find yourself on the ground with an attacker on top of you, your goal is to regain control. Use your legs to "bridge" your hips upward, which can momentarily disrupt their balance.

Simultaneously drop the leg that you are going to be going in the direction of and roll out. You will also end up on the floor but in a better position than on your back. Scramble to get up quickly while continuing to strike vulnerable areas until you can escape.

Ponytail Grab

If someone grabs your hair, resist the urge to pull away directly, as this will only increase the pain and allow them to control your movement. Instead, grab their wrist with both hands to reduce the tension on your scalp. Step toward them, not away, which will lessen their leverage. Once close enough, use a distraction technique such as shin kick or a foot stomp, then rotate your body out of the grip to escape.

PRACTICAL TRAINING EXERCISES FOR WOMEN

Practical training exercises are a crucial component of any self-defence program, especially for women who want to develop the skills and confidence needed to protect themselves effectively.

Exercises such as partner drills, role-playing scenarios, strength and conditioning exercises, and mental training will help focus on building muscle memory, enhancing physical fitness, and simulating real-life scenarios to ensure readiness in the face of potential threats.

By engaging in consistent and structured training, you can transform the theoretical knowledge into instinctive actions, empowering you to respond decisively and effectively when your safety is at risk. You will no longer have to worry whether you will fight or freeze – you will be prepared to fight!

LEGAL IMPLICATIONS OF SELF-DEFENCE

My first recommendation when it comes to the legal implications of personal defence strategies is to be sure you know and understand your own local and provincial/state laws. Obviously, I can't address the laws that pertain to every geographical area, but I have a general understanding of what you should be aware of should you find yourself in a scenario where you might have to get physical to protect yourself.

Most jurisdictions allow the use of reasonable force to protect oneself from harm. This means using only as much force as necessary to stop the threat. Once the threat is stopped, you must cease all force.

No matter the circumstances surrounding the attack or threat, it's crucial to report any self-defence incident to the police immediately and provide a clear and honest account of what happened. If feasible, collect any contact information from any independent witnesses who can corroborate your account of the event. If any injuries were sustained as a result of the incident, keep medical records as documentation and evidence.

Always be able to articulate why the use of force was necessary, emphasizing the immediate threat to personal safety. Demonstrate that the force used was proportional to the threat faced.

You can always consult with a lawyer who can help you navigate through any potential legal consequences and ensure one's rights are protected.

Darun's Story

I was once teaching a self-defence class to a group of women and I was so inspired by a friend's story. Her name is Darun and her story gave me chills. Here is what she shared on social media:

> On September 15th at 11:00 A.M. at Massey Park in Brampton, a predator attacked me in the one space I felt most peaceful.
>
> I saw him walking with his bike 10 minutes before the attack.
>
> He hid his bike in the woods and

approached me from behind. Thank God I turned around the second I did because his intentions were to attack from behind.

I caught him off guard when I turned around and he got nervous... took off his face mask and asked me for my YouTube handle. I told him I wasn't giving him any of my information.

He put his mask back on, looked at my tripod to see if it was recording, looked around to see if there were people and then looked me dead in the eye with the craziest look I've ever gotten from another human.

He then charged towards me and raised his hands towards my throat... and before he could get to me I punched him as hard as I could in his jaw.

He was shocked for a split second and then grabbed me and I continued to fight.

My voice finally came through and I screamed for help when I realized he was looking for something to hit me with.

The cops were called the same time I started screaming for help by a witness who heard me scream and the police showed up minutes after.

He planned my attack.

He dressed for it.

He just picked the wrong victim.

Because I am here to raise hell.
And I am not going to be silent about it.
I am sick and tired of women living in fear.

This is why we clench our keys in between our fingers.

This is why the whole squad won't fall asleep until everyone in the group chat says they got home safe.

I shouldn't have to hear that I 'shouldn't have been out there alone at 11:00 A.M.' in a public space, in the middle of the day.

I loved hearing this story at our self-defence workshop. Her vulnerability was so appreciated by everyone there. It brought a rawness and realness to the topics we were talking about. Most people will never experience a situation like that in their life but to know it can happen anywhere and at any time really brought things into perspective. Standing your ground, being assertive, and relying on your training really helps.

·

CHAPTER 6

SAFETY MEASURES FOR TRAVELING ALONE

Have you ever traveled alone, or does the thought of it scare you?

Traveling alone can be an incredibly empowering and enriching experience, offering the freedom to explore new places on your own terms. However, solo travel also comes with unique safety challenges that require careful planning and vigilance. This chapter will cover essential safety measures for women traveling alone, focusing on preparing for solo trips, choosing safe accommodations, and planning for emergencies.

After reading these guidelines, you can not only enhance your personal safety, but enjoy your solo adventures with greater confidence and peace of mind!

PREPARING FOR SOLO TRIPS - CONSIDERATIONS

Research Your Destination

Understand the cultural norms, laws, and societal expectations of your destination. This knowledge will help you avoid inadvertently offending locals or violating laws, and it will guide your behaviour to align with local customs.

Research the safety conditions of the destination, including crime rates, areas to avoid, and common scams targeting tourists. Government travel advisories and traveler forums are excellent resources for this information. Google is your best friend!

Health and Travel Insurance

Check if any vaccinations are required or recommended for your destination. Carry a basic medical kit with essentials like pain relievers, antiseptics, and any prescription medications you may need.

Purchase comprehensive travel insurance that covers medical emergencies, trip cancellations, lost luggage, and theft. Ensure your insurance policy includes coverage for solo travellers and any adventurous activities you plan to undertake.

Planning Your Itinerary

Plan your itinerary in detail, including transportation schedules, accommodation addresses, and points of interest. Share your itinerary with a trusted friend or family member back home. Always have a contingency plan in place for unexpected changes or emergencies, such as knowing the location of the nearest embassy or consulate and having alternate accommodation options.

Packing Essentials

Carry personal safety items like a personal alarm, whistle, or pepper spray (where legally permitted) for added security. A portable doorstop alarm can also be useful for securing your hotel room. Pack a universal adapter, a portable charger, and a money belt or hidden pouch for valuables.

Digital Considerations

Ensure your phone is unlocked for international use or purchase a local SIM card upon arrival. Download essential travel apps, including maps, translation services, and emergency contact apps. Protect your digital information by using VPNs on public Wi-Fi networks and being cautious about sharing personal details on social media. Do not post in real time!

Safe Accommodation Choices

Choosing safe accommodations is a crucial aspect of traveling, especially for women who are exploring new destinations alone. Where you stay can significantly impact your overall safety and peace of mind during your trip. From selecting reputable hotels to ensuring secure rental options, making informed decisions about your lodging can help mitigate risks and provide a secure base from which to explore.

Research and Reviews

Always use reputable travel websites to read reviews from other solo female travellers about potential accommodations. Pay attention to comments on safety, cleanliness, and staff behaviour. Ensure your accommodation is in a safe neighbourhood with easy access to transportation, restaurants, and emergency services.

Choose the Right Type of Accommodation

Hotels often offer more security features, such as 24-hour reception and in-room safes. Hostels can be safe and social but choose those with female-only dorms and secure storage facilities.

If opting for a rental such as an Airbnb, verify the host's identity and read reviews carefully. Look for properties with strong security measures, such as secure locks and well-lit entrances.

Security Features

When booking, inquire about the security features of your room, such as deadbolts, peepholes, and secure windows. Avoid rooms on the ground floor as they can be more accessible to intruders. Choose accommodations with security cameras and on-site security personnel.

Arrival and Check-In

Arrive and check into your accommodation during the day if possible to familiarize yourself with the surroundings and address any concerns with the staff. Note the location of the reception desk and emergency exits. Make sure the staff is aware that you are traveling alone for additional support if needed.

During Your Stay

Keep your accommodation details private. Avoid disclosing your room number and travel plans to strangers. Have local emergency numbers and the contact information of your accommodation handy. Know how to contact the front desk quickly in case of an emergency.

Emergency Response Planning

When traveling, particularly as a solo female traveler, having a well-thought-out emergency response plan is essential for maintaining safety and peace of mind. Unexpected situations, from medical emergencies to lost belongings or sudden changes in local conditions, can arise without warning. Being prepared with a comprehensive emergency plan ensures that you can handle these situations effectively and minimize potential risks.

Identifying Emergency Resources

Familiarize yourself with the local emergency numbers, including police, fire, and medical services. In many countries, these numbers differ from those in your home country. Know the location and contact information of your country's embassy or consulate. They can provide assistance in case of legal issues, lost passports, or emergencies.

Emergency Contacts

Maintain regular contact with a trusted friend or family member. Share your itinerary and check in at agreed intervals. If possible, establish a local contact, such as a tour guide or a friend, who can assist you in emergencies.

Emergency Kits

Carry a comprehensive medical kit, including any prescription medications, bandages, antiseptics, and over-the-counter medications for common ailments. Have a backup of essential documents (passport, insurance, visas) in both physical and digital forms. Keep a small amount of emergency cash in a separate location from your main wallet.

Personal Safety Strategies

Consider taking a self-defence course before your trip to build confidence and learn practical techniques as discussed in Chapter 5 for protecting yourself. Always stay alert to your surroundings, especially in unfamiliar or crowded places. Avoid distractions like excessive phone use, and trust your instincts if something feels off.

———

While it's undeniably more pleasant and far less stressful to focus solely on the excitement and joy of a holiday or vacation, the reality is that unexpected situations can arise, regardless of whether you're traveling alone or with others. It's natural to want to avoid thinking about the potential for things to go awry, but taking the time to prepare in advance is crucial.

Being well-prepared equips you to handle emergencies, danger, or other challenging circumstances more effectively. This foresight not only enhances your personal safety but also empowers you to enjoy your travels with greater peace of mind.

Whether you're venturing into far-off, unfamiliar territories or simply stepping out of your geographical comfort zone, proactive planning and awareness can make all the difference. By embracing a mindset of readiness and vigilance, you can navigate your journeys with confidence, knowing that you are equipped to protect yourself and respond to any situation that may arise.

Remember, your safety is paramount, and taking these small but important steps proactively ensures that your adventures remain as enjoyable and worry-free as possible.

CHAPTER 7

CYBERSECURITY AND ONLINE SAFETY

The internet is an undeniable part of our daily lives, and I don't see that changing anytime soon. It offers countless opportunities for communication, education, and entertainment. However, with these benefits come significant risks, especially for women who are often targeted by cybercriminals and online predators.

As we navigate the digital world, it is crucial to be aware of the potential dangers and take proactive steps to protect ourselves. This chapter will explore why we need to be mindful of our safety online; the dangers of online insecurity; and provide practical advice on safeguarding personal information online, securing social media accounts, and recognizing online threats.

By understanding and implementing these strategies, women can enjoy the advantages of the digital age while minimizing the risks and maintaining their safety and privacy.

WHY WE NEED TO BE MINDFUL OF OUR SAFETY ONLINE

In today's digital age, women face unique cybersecurity challenges that require vigilance and proactive measures. Cyber threats can take many forms, including phishing scams, identity theft, online harassment, and cyberstalking.

Understanding these threats is the first step towards protecting oneself. Phishing scams often involve deceptive emails or messages that trick individuals into divulging personal information. Identity theft can result from data breaches or unsecured online activities, leading to significant financial and emotional distress.

Online harassment and cyberstalking are particularly concerning, as they can escalate into real-world threats. Recognizing these risks and understanding how they manifest is crucial for implementing effective online safety practices.

———

Case Study: Hidden Internet Dangers

Consider the case of Roxanne, a university student who fell victim to a phishing scam she was unaware of and unprepared for.

Like many students, Roxanne was mindful of her finances, diligently saving her earnings to support her education and daily expenses. One evening, after a long day of classes and work, she received an email that appeared to be from her bank. The email carried an urgent tone, stating that her account needed immediate verification to avoid being frozen.

The email looked professional, adorned with the bank's logo and official-sounding language. Exhausted and caught off guard, Roxanne trusted the legitimacy of the message. She clicked on the provided link and was directed to a website that looked identical to her bank's official site. Without a second thought, she entered her personal information, including her banking credentials, and submitted the form, feeling relieved that she had addressed the issue promptly.

Within hours, Roxanne's relief turned into a nightmare. Her bank account was drained, and she began receiving alerts for transactions she hadn't made. Panic set in as she realized that her personal information had been compromised. The fraudulent website had been a meticulously crafted phishing scam, designed to deceive unsuspecting individuals like Roxanne into divulging sensitive information.

The aftermath was overwhelming. Not only did Roxanne lose her hard-earned savings, but her personal information was also sold on the dark web, exposing her to further risks of identity theft. The financial loss was devastating, but the emotional toll was equally significant. Roxanne spent months dealing with the repercussions, including the stress of recovering her stolen funds, securing her personal information, and restoring her credit. This ordeal affected her studies and well-being, casting a shadow over her once bright and hopeful university experience.

Roxanne's story is a stark reminder of how easily one can fall prey to online scams and the severe consequences that follow. Her experience underscores the importance of vigilance and skepticism when dealing with unsolicited communications, especially those requesting personal information. By sharing her story, we can learn valuable lessons about protecting ourselves in the digital age, emphasizing the need for caution and awareness to safeguard our personal and financial security.

SECURING PERSONAL INFORMATION ONLINE

Strong Passwords

Create strong, unique passwords for each online account. A strong password typically includes a mix of upper and lower case letters, numbers, and special characters. Avoid using easily guessable information, such as birthdays or pet names. Consider using a password manager to securely store and manage your passwords.

Two-Factor Authentication (2FA)

Enable two-factor authentication wherever possible. 2FA adds an extra layer of security by requiring not only a password but also a second form of verification, such as a text message code or an authentication app. This makes it significantly harder for cybercriminals to gain access to your accounts.

Secure Connections

Always use secure, encrypted connections when accessing sensitive information online. Look for "https://" in the URL and a padlock symbol in the browser address bar. Avoid using public Wi-Fi networks for online banking or shopping, as these networks are often less secure.

Regular Updates

Keep your software and devices up to date with the latest security patches and updates. Cybercriminals often exploit vulnerabilities in outdated software to gain access to personal information. Regular updates help protect against these threats.

Personal Information Sharing

Be mindful of the personal information you share online. Limit the details you post on social media and other platforms, and adjust privacy settings to control who can see your information. Avoid sharing sensitive information, such as your full address or phone number, publicly.

SOCIAL MEDIA PRIVACY AND SECURITY

In our increasingly more digital and interconnected world, social media has become such a powerful tool for connection and self-expression. However, it also presents unique risks, especially for women who need to be vigilant about their privacy and security online.

There are some essential strategies for safeguarding your personal information on social media platforms that I'd like to highlight here. From fine-tuning your privacy settings to being cautious about who you connect with, these practices are crucial for maintaining control over your digital presence and ensuring your safety in a world where oversharing can have serious consequences.

Privacy Settings

Review and adjust the privacy settings on your social media accounts to control who can see your posts and personal information. Limit your audience to trusted friends and family, and avoid making sensitive information publicly accessible.

Be Selective with Connections

Only accept friend requests and connection invitations from people you know and trust. Cybercriminals often create fake profiles to gather personal information or perpetrate scams. Verify the identity of anyone who sends you a request before accepting it.

Monitor Your Digital Footprint

Regularly review the information available about you online. Search your name to see what information appears in search results and take steps to remove or secure any sensitive data. This can help prevent identity theft and protect your reputation.

Oversharing

Be cautious about the information you share on social media. Avoid posting real-time updates about your location, vacation plans, or other personal details that could be used to track or harm you. Share such information with a trusted circle of friends and family only.

Report and Block Abusers

If you encounter harassment or abuse on social media, use the platform's tools to report and block the abuser. Most social media sites have mechanisms in place to handle harassment and protect users. Take advantage of these tools to maintain a safe online environment.

RECOGNIZING ONLINE THREATS AND SCAMS

Now more than ever before, the internet seems to have become a complex and sneaky breeding ground for sophisticated scams and online threats that can compromise your personal security. Women, in particular, are often targeted by cybercriminals who use cunning tactics to exploit trust and gain access to sensitive information. The following section explores common online threats, from phishing scams to fake websites, and provides crucial tips for recognizing and avoiding these dangers. By staying informed and vigilant, you can protect yourself from falling victim to these malicious schemes and maintain control over your digital life.

Phishing Scams

Phishing scams involve fraudulent messages that appear to be from legitimate sources, such as banks or social media platforms, designed to trick you into revealing personal information. Be wary of unsolicited emails, texts, or messages asking for sensitive information. Verify the legitimacy of the sender before responding.

Fake Websites

Cybercriminals often create fake websites that mimic legitimate ones to steal your information. Before entering any personal or financial information, check the URL for accuracy and look for indicators of security, such as "https://" and a padlock symbol.

Malware and Ransomware

Malware and ransomware are malicious software designed to damage or control your device. Avoid downloading attachments or clicking on links from unknown or suspicious sources. Install reputable antivirus software and keep it updated to protect against these threats.

Social Engineering

Social engineering involves manipulating individuals into divulging confidential information. Be cautious of unsolicited requests for information or attempts to gain your trust quickly. Verify the identity of anyone asking for personal details and be skeptical of unexpected requests.

Scams Targeting Women

Be aware of scams that specifically target women, such as romance scams, where perpetrators build fake relationships to extract money or personal information. Stay vigilant and look for warning signs, such as requests for money, overly flattering communication, or inconsistencies in their stories.

———

It is important to be mindful of the dangers that can threaten your safety, whether you're entering an experience in real life, or online. Unfortunately, there are people out there who prey on people making haphazard decisions by trusting things that may look legitimate but aren't. It can be difficult to decipher truth from fiction in our ever-evolving digital world, so it's important to build your digital proficiency muscles and practice self-awareness as it pertains to your digital presence.

CHAPTER 8

BUILDING A SAFETY SUPPORT NETWORK

There is a scene in the popular HBO series Girls[1] where the oblivious and innocent main character, Hannah, is picked up on the side of the road by a man offering her a ride and she takes it without considering the risks.

Partway through the drive, she notices some questionable behaviours and red flags from the man who is driving – a visible weapon in the back seat, a car full of bags and belongings, some strange phrases from the man, among other things. When she realizes she could be in real danger after making such a poor judgement call, she makes a phone call to her friend Marnie and begins casually describing the man she's with, his age, appearance, the car they're in and where exactly they are on the route.

Quickly, Marnie realizes what is happening and starts asking Hannah yes or no questions, so as to not make the driver aware of what Hannah is doing. When she realizes – because Hannah and Marnie have clearly practised or discussed this procedure at length in advance – she first asks, "Is this a safety call?" so that Hannah can easily say "Mmhmm! Yup!" without having to explain anything or share that she feels unsafe.

In this scenario, Marnie and Hannah have prepped in advance about what to do if a "Safety Call" situation happens. They are both well aware of what info to share or ask, how to behave and act, and how to offer support for the other person to ensure that she is going to have the best chances of being safe and sound in the near future.

This scenario is all too real for many women. The feeling of vulnerability can strike at any time, but having a trusted safety support network and an emergency procedure for unsafe or vulnerable situations can turn fear into empowerment. Whether it's a friend who knows your daily routine, a family member who tracks your location when you're out late, a community group that shares safety tips, or a prepared and practised "safety call" procedure for unsafe situations that arise, these connections are crucial. In this chapter, we'll explore how to build a robust safety support network that you can rely on in moments of uncertainty, ensuring that you're never truly alone, no matter the situation.

Building a safety support network significantly enhances a woman's ability to navigate various life situations with confidence and security. This network is comprised of trusted individuals, community resources, and strategic plans that work together to provide emotional support, practical assistance, and valuable information.

In this chapter, we will identify trusted contacts, how to communicate safety plans with family and friends, and how to utilize community resources to establish a comprehensive and effective safety support network.

IDENTIFYING TRUSTED CONTACTS

Identifying trusted contacts begins with evaluating the trustworthiness of individuals in your circle. Trustworthy people are those who demonstrate reliability, integrity, and consistency in their actions and words. These individuals can include family members, close friends, and co-workers who have shown they are dependable in both everyday and emergency situations. Trustworthy contacts are not only loyal, but should also respect your boundaries, maintain confidentiality, and support your overall well-being.

Family and Friends

Start by considering those closest to you, such as family and friends, who have a vested interest in your safety. These individuals are often the cornerstone of your support network due to their emotional investment and familiarity with your life circumstances. Establish open lines of communication with them about your safety concerns and plans, ensuring they understand their role in your support network. These are often people who you have a "safe word" with.

Work and Community Contacts

Once you have your family and friends secured as trusted contacts, you can then expand your network to include co-workers, neighbours, and certain community members. These individuals can provide additional support, especially when family and close friends are not immediately available. These trusted contacts are usually actively involved in local safety initiatives or community groups, which indicates a commitment to community well-being.

Building New Connections

You can then actively seek out new connections through social events, community groups, and online forums that align with your interests and values. Volunteering, joining sports clubs, or participating in hobby groups can help you meet like-minded individuals who can become part of your safety network. Be cautious with online connections, verifying the authenticity and trustworthiness of individuals before incorporating them into your network.

COMMUNICATING SAFETY PLANS WITH FAMILY AND FRIENDS

Effectively communicating your safety plans with family and friends is crucial to ensuring their support and involvement. Clear communication helps them understand your needs, recognize potential threats, and respond appropriately in case of an emergency. It also fosters a sense of accountability and ensures that someone knows your whereabouts and plans.

Sharing Your Plans

Inform your trusted contacts about your travel itineraries, daily routines, and any changes in your schedule. Sharing this information allows them to monitor your safety and provide help if necessary. Make sure they know your emergency contacts, medical information, and any specific instructions for different scenarios.

Establish Regular Check-Ins

Regular check-ins are paramount in maintaining a safety support network. Establish a routine for checking in with key members of your network, whether daily, weekly, or before and after specific activities.

These check-ins can be as simple as a text message, phone call, or an update through a messaging app. Regular communication helps to alert your network if something goes wrong and ensures they can take prompt action if needed.

Utilizing Technology for Communication

Leverage technology to facilitate communication and enhance your safety network. Group chats on messaging apps can be an efficient way to keep everyone updated simultaneously.

Use location-sharing apps like "Find My Friends" to allow trusted individuals to track your whereabouts in real-time. Ensure that everyone in your network is familiar with these tools and knows how to use them effectively.

Creating Emergency Plans

Develop and communicate detailed emergency plans for various scenarios, such as getting lost, encountering a threat, or facing a medical emergency.

Outline specific steps for each situation, including who to contact, where to go, and what actions to take. Make sure your network understands these plans and their respective roles in executing them.

UTILIZING COMMUNITY RESOURCES

Law Enforcement and Emergency Services

Familiarize yourself and establish a relationship with local law enforcement and emergency services. Know the contact information for non-emergency situations and understand how to report suspicious activities.

Many police departments offer community outreach programs, safety workshops, and resources specifically for women. Attend these programs to build a rapport with local officers and gain insights into local safety concerns.

Local Organizations

Women's shelters, crisis centres, and community organizations are valuable resources that can enhance your safety support network. They provide immediate safety, support services, and advocacy for women facing violence or abuse. These organizations often offer counselling, legal assistance, and emergency housing, which can be crucial during a crisis.

Educational Institutions

Utilize the safety resources provided by your educational institution. Campus security services often include personal escort services, emergency call boxes, and safety apps designed to protect students. Participate in any available self-defence classes, safety workshops, and support groups to enhance your knowledge and skills.

Public Resources

Libraries, community centres, and public spaces frequently host safety events, workshops, and provide information on local resources. These venues are also excellent places to meet people and expand your support network. Public transportation systems often have safety features such as emergency contacts, safe waiting areas, and security personnel. Familiarize yourself with these features to enhance your safety while commuting.

Online Resources

Leverage online resources to stay informed about safety tips, self-defence techniques, and local safety issues. Many websites, forums, and social media groups focus on women's safety, providing a platform for sharing experiences, advice, and support. Ensure you verify the credibility of these sources and be cautious when sharing personal information online.

Keep your safety support network close and ensure you maintain and strengthen this network through regular communication, mutual support, and continuous education to ensure that your network remains well-protected and confident.

Do you have a safety support network?

If not, think about who in your existing circle could be involved in yours, and reach out to them in order to discuss next steps for having plans in place for safety procedures in the future.

---

1. *Girls*. Season 3, Episode 6, "Free Snacks." Directed by Richard Shepard. Written by Lena Dunham. Aired February 9, 2014, on HBO.

CHAPTER 9

EMPOWERING YOU TO TAKE CHARGE OF YOUR SAFETY

As we get near to the end of the book, I want you to start thinking about taking charge of your own safety. I want to empower you to take charge of your personal safety as it is a fundamental step towards living confidently and securely.

As you have read in the previous chapters, women's safety is not just about physical protection but also encompasses emotional, psychological, and digital security. In this chapter I want to summarize some points I have previously talked about, and delve into three critical areas: Taking Control of Your Environment, Risk Assessment and Mitigation Strategies, and Encouraging Independence and Vigilance.

TAKING CONTROL OF YOUR ENVIRONMENT

Taking control of your environment means creating a safe and secure space wherever you are. This involves being aware of your surroundings, making informed decisions about your living and working spaces, and utilizing tools and strategies to enhance your safety.

HOME SAFETY

Locks and Alarms

Ensure that your home is equipped with sturdy locks on all doors and windows. Consider installing a security system with alarms and surveillance cameras. Smart home devices, such as doorbell cameras and motion sensors can provide additional layers of security.

Lighting

Adequate lighting is crucial for home safety. Install outdoor lighting around entry points and pathways to deter intruders. Inside, ensure that all areas are well-lit, particularly entrances, stairways, and hallways.

Emergency Plan

A must! Develop and regularly update an emergency plan. This should include escape routes, designated safe rooms, and emergency contact numbers. Practice the plan with all household members to ensure everyone knows what to do in case of an emergency.

WORKPLACE SAFETY

Awareness

Stay aware of your surroundings in the workplace. Know the layout of your building, including exits and emergency equipment locations. Familiarize yourself with the company's safety policies and procedures.

Personal Belongings

Keep personal belongings secure. Use a lockable drawer or locker for valuables and sensitive documents. Be cautious about leaving personal items unattended.

Safety Measures

Ensure there are safety measures in your workplace. This could include requesting security patrols, improved lighting in parking areas, and access to self-defence training or safety workshops.

PUBLIC SPACES

There are a few things to keep in mind when it comes to maintaining your safety while out in public spaces.

Vigilance

Maintain a high level of awareness in public spaces. Avoid distractions such as using your phone or wearing headphones while walking. Stay alert to your surroundings and trust your instincts.

Safe Routes

Plan your routes in advance and choose well-lit, populated paths. If possible, walk with a companion, especially at night. If you feel uncomfortable, find a safe place, such as a store or a crowded area.

Public Transportation

When using public transportation, sit near the driver or in populated areas of the vehicle. Keep your personal belongings close and be mindful of your surroundings. If you feel unsafe, alert the driver or conductor.

RISK ASSESSMENT AND MITIGATION STRATEGIES

Risk assessment and mitigation are proactive steps to identify potential threats and develop strategies to minimize their impact. This approach empowers women to anticipate dangers and respond effectively.

IDENTIFYING RISKS

Personal Risk Factors

Assess your personal risk factors based on your lifestyle, daily routines, and the environments you frequent. Consider factors such as the time of day you travel, the areas you visit, and any patterns that could make you a target.

Environmental Risks

Evaluate the safety of your home, workplace, and the public spaces you frequent. Look for potential vulnerabilities, such as poorly lit areas, unsecured entrances, or lack of security measures.

MITIGATION STRATEGIES

Self-Defence Training

Enrol in self-defence classes to learn techniques for protecting yourself. These classes not only teach physical defence skills but also boost confidence and awareness.

Safety Apps

Utilize safety apps on your smartphone. Apps like bSafe, Noonlight, and Circle of 6 provide features such as location tracking, emergency alerts, and instant connection to emergency contacts.

Safety Network

Establish a network of trusted individuals who can support you in emergencies. Share your travel plans and check-in regularly with family or friends.

EMERGENCY PREPAREDNESS

Emergency Kit

Prepare an emergency kit with essentials such as a flashlight, first aid supplies, a whistle, and a portable phone charger. Keep this kit in an easily accessible location.

Communication Plan

Develop a communication plan with your emergency contacts. Ensure everyone knows how to reach each other in case of an emergency and establish a meeting point if you are separated.

Regular Drills

Practice emergency drills regularly. This includes fire drills, evacuation plans, and lockdown procedures. Familiarity with these procedures can save valuable time in a real emergency.

ENCOURAGING INDEPENDENCE AND VIGILANCE

Encouraging independence and vigilance involves a mindset of proactive awareness by staying informed, confident, and prepared.

BUILDING CONFIDENCE

Education and Training

Invest in education and training to build confidence in your ability to protect yourself. This includes self-defence classes, safety workshops, and learning about personal security measures.

Assertiveness

Develop assertiveness skills to confidently set boundaries and stand up for yourself. Practice clear communication and the ability to say no when necessary.

Self-Reliance

Develop practical skills such as basic first aid, car maintenance, and navigation. These skills enhance your ability to handle unexpected situations independently.

STAY INFORMED

Current Issues

Stay informed about current threats and safety issues in your area. Follow local news, community alerts, and online safety resources to keep up-to-date with potential risks.

Safety Resources

Utilize available safety resources such as local police departments, community organizations, and online forums. These resources provide valuable information and support for personal safety.

Networking

Build a network of supportive individuals who share your commitment to safety. Participate in community groups, attend safety workshops, and engage with online communities focused on women's safety.

PRACTICE VIGILANCE

Awareness

Maintain a heightened sense of awareness in all situations. This includes being mindful of your surroundings, recognizing potential threats, and trusting your instincts.

Routine Checks

Incorporate routine safety checks into your daily habits. This includes checking locks, ensuring your phone is charged, and reviewing emergency plans regularly.

Preparedness

Stay prepared for unexpected situations by carrying essential items such as a whistle, personal alarm, and any self-defence items (where applicable – check local laws). Knowing you have these tools at your disposal can increase your sense of security.

———

Take a moment to reflect on everything we've covered about taking control of your own safety. Just like a captain steering a ship through unpredictable waters, your personal safety is in your hands. It's about understanding your environment, assessing risks, and being prepared for whatever comes your way.

Taking charge of your safety isn't about living in fear; it's about living with confidence. Imagine walking into a room where you know the exits, understand your surroundings, and feel empowered by the knowledge you carry. It's like when you're packing for a long trip; you wouldn't leave without essentials like your passport or a map. Similarly, in life, you shouldn't go without the tools and awareness that make you feel secure.

I think about a story I once heard about a woman who, after being stranded during a trip, learned the importance of always having a "Plan B." She made sure that from then on, she had backups for her backups—spare phone chargers, emergency contacts, and even an extra pair of shoes. It may seem like a small thing, but the peace of mind it gave her was life-changing. That's what preparedness does: *it helps you feel in control, even when things don't go according to plan.*

In the same way, you've got the power to navigate the challenges and uncertainties life may present. Whether it's understanding the safety features in your home, being aware of your surroundings in public, or having the confidence to assert your boundaries, you're building layers of protection for yourself.

Remember, this isn't just about reacting to danger – it's about proactively shaping a life where you feel safe, capable, and confident in every space you enter. You're the captain of your ship, and no matter what waters you sail through, you've got the strength, knowledge, and tools to guide you safely to shore.

CHAPTER 10

COPING WITH TRAUMA

Trauma is an emotional response to a distressing event or series of events that can have long-lasting effects on an individual's mental and physical well-being.

For women, trauma can stem from various sources, including violence, abuse, accidents, significant life changes, and more. Understanding trauma, recognizing its signs, seeking help, and developing resilience are crucial steps in the journey toward recovery. This last chapter aims to provide a comprehensive guide on coping with trauma, focusing on the types of trauma, recognizing signs, seeking counselling, and building resilience.

A friend of mine once shared a story with me about something that happened to her that didn't seem like a big deal at the time, but it ended up affecting many areas of her life in ways she never expected.

She loved jogging early in the morning, right as the sun was coming up. It was her time to clear her mind and start the day on a positive note. One morning, though, as she was nearing the end of her usual route, a car slowed down beside her.

The driver rolled down the window and started making inappropriate comments. It was a male driver in a dark vehicle; he was wearing dark clothing and a hooded sweatshirt that shadowed much of his face. He was making threatening and dangerous comments, alluding to the fact that a woman could easily be "snatched up" if she isn't careful running alone in a secluded place.

Understandably, she immediately felt a rush of fear, insecurity, and stress, but she tried to brush it off and pick up her pace until she could access a walking path nearby that wasn't accessible by car.

Eventually, she was out of immediate harm, and continued her run despite the additional anxiety and pending threat to her safety. She made it home safely, called her mom to tell her what had transpired, and carried on with the rest of her day.

She didn't think much of it afterward and didn't tell anyone else, convincing herself that it was just a random, one-off encounter. She knew she was now safe, but she also made some accommodations to her exercise plan in order to feel more confident and calm while working out. She joined a public gym facility temporarily so she could do her run without feeling afraid of potential strangers, and learned safety preparedness just to be sure that she felt safer on the next run she tried outdoors.

Despite all of this, over the next few days, she started to notice some changes in herself. She became hyper-aware of her surroundings, constantly on edge even in places that had always felt safe. Even walking outside in open areas suddenly felt dangerous and she felt unable to go outside for long stretches of time in public places.

Every car that passed made her heart race, and she found herself looking over her shoulder more often than not. She avoided the route where the incident happened and then, bit by bit, stopped jogging outside completely. What seemed like a small incident had taken away something she loved.

It didn't stop there, either. She found herself replaying the moment in her head at the most unexpected times – at work during important tasks, when she was supposed to be relaxing, and even when she was trying to fall asleep. She began to feel uneasy and guilty, questioning whether she had handled the situation properly and stressing about how it was her own fault for taking that particular route and going at that particular time.

Chronic feelings of self-doubt started creeping into other parts of her life, making her more stressed and irritable. Even her daily decisions were affected. Simple choices, like where to park or which streets to walk down, became sources of anxiety. What had once been her sense of safety now felt fragile and easily shattered. This one "little" experience with danger started permeating every thought and action she was taking, and this lasted for months.

Talking with her made me realize how something that seems minor can have a profound impact. It wasn't until she recognized these changes and started seeking support that she began to rebuild her sense of safety and control. It's a reminder that even the "little" traumas can ripple through our lives in unexpected ways, and it's important to acknowledge their effects and seek help when needed.

TYPES OF TRAUMA

Acute Trauma

Acute trauma results from a single stressful or dangerous event, such as a car accident, natural disaster, or sudden loss of a loved one. The intensity of the event leads to immediate and severe emotional reactions.

Chronic Trauma

Chronic trauma is a type that occurs from repeated and prolonged exposure to highly stressful events. Examples include ongoing domestic violence, long-term child abuse, or enduring bullying.

Secondary Trauma

This type of trauma occurs when an individual is exposed to the trauma of others. It is common among professionals who work with trauma survivors, such as social workers, therapists, and emergency responders.

Developmental Trauma

Developmental trauma refers to exposure to early life trauma, including abuse, neglect, and disrupted attachment relationships during critical developmental periods. It can lead to long-term difficulties in emotional regulation, cognition, and behaviour.

The impact of trauma, whether from a seemingly minor incident or a major event, can ripple through every aspect of a woman's life in unexpected and profound ways. As illustrated through the story shared, what may appear as a "small" incident can fundamentally alter one's sense of safety, daily routines, and emotional well-being.

Understanding that trauma manifests differently for everyone — whether acute, chronic, developmental, or secondary — is crucial for both prevention and healing.

This chapter serves as a reminder that no traumatic experience should be minimized, and seeking support is not only acceptable but essential for recovery. By recognizing the signs of trauma, acknowledging its effects, and actively pursuing help, women can begin to rebuild their sense of safety and control.

Remember, the journey to healing is personal, and taking steps to protect both your physical and emotional well-being is an integral part of self-defence and personal safety.

RECOGNIZING SIGNS OF TRAUMA

Recognizing the signs of trauma is the first step toward seeking help and beginning the healing process. Trauma manifests in a variety of emotional, psychological, and physical symptoms, which can differ from person to person.

EMOTIONAL AND PSYCHOLOGICAL SIGNS

Anxiety and Fear

Persistent feelings of anxiety and fear are common, often triggered by reminders of the traumatic event.

Depression

Feelings of sadness, hopelessness, and a lack of interest in previously enjoyable activities can indicate trauma.

Flashbacks and Nightmares

Re-experiencing the traumatic event through flashbacks and nightmares is a hallmark symptom of trauma.

Irritability and Anger

Increased irritability and anger, often over minor issues, can be a sign of unresolved trauma.

Emotional Numbness

Difficulty in experiencing positive emotions and a general sense of emotional numbness can occur.

Hyper-vigilance

Being constantly on edge, easily startled, and overly aware of potential dangers.

PHYSICAL SIGNS

Fatigue

Chronic fatigue and exhaustion are common, even with adequate rest.

Sleep Disturbances

Difficulty falling or staying asleep, frequent nightmares, or insomnia.

Physical Aches and Pains

Unexplained physical symptoms such as headaches, stomachaches, and muscle tension.

Changes in Appetite

Significant changes in eating habits, including loss of appetite or overeating.

Increased Heart Rate and Sweating

Physical responses to stress, such as increased heart rate and sweating, even in non-threatening situations.

SEEKING HELP AND COUNSELLING

Seeking help and counselling is a vital step in the recovery process from trauma. Professional support can provide the necessary tools and techniques to process and heal from traumatic experiences. Seeking help is a courageous step towards healing. Professional support can provide invaluable guidance and strategies to manage and overcome the effects of trauma.

TYPES OF PROFESSIONAL HELP

Therapists and Counsellors

Licensed professionals trained in trauma-specific therapies, such as cognitive-behavioural therapy (CBT), eye movement desensitization and reprocessing (EMDR), and dialectical behaviour therapy (DBT).

Support Groups

Groups led by trained facilitators that offer a safe space for individuals to share experiences and support each other.

Psychiatrists

Medical doctors who can prescribe medication to help manage symptoms of trauma, such as anxiety and depression.

FINDING THE RIGHT THERAPIST

It is so important to find the right therapist for you. Here are some of the things to look out for when seeking out the help of a therapist

Credentials and Specialization

Look for therapists who are licensed and have specialized training in trauma-focused therapies.

Comfort and Trust

It's so important to feel comfortable and build trust with your therapist. If you don't feel a connection, it's okay to seek another professional.

Recommendations and Reviews

Ask for recommendations from trusted sources or look for reviews online to find reputable professionals.

WHAT TO EXPECT IN THERAPY

Initial Assessment

The therapist will conduct an initial assessment to understand your history, symptoms, and specific needs.

Goal Setting

You will both set goals for what you want to achieve in therapy.

Therapeutic Techniques

The therapist will use various techniques tailored to your needs, such as exposure therapy, cognitive restructuring, and relaxation techniques to help you achieve your goals.

Progress Monitoring

Regularly reviewing progress and making adjustments to the treatment plan as needed.

BUILDING RESILIENCE AND RECOVERY STRATEGIES

Building resilience and developing recovery strategies are essential for long-term healing and well-being. Resilience involves the ability to bounce back from adversity and grow stronger through the recovery process.

DEVELOPING RESILIENCE

Self-Care

Prioritize self-care activities that promote physical, emotional, and mental well-being. This includes regular exercise, healthy eating, sufficient sleep, and engaging in hobbies and activities that bring you happiness..

Mindfulness and Relaxation

Practice mindfulness techniques such as meditation, deep breathing, and progressive muscle relaxation to reduce stress and enhance emotional regulation.

Positive and Nurturing Relationships

Build and maintain supportive relationships with family, friends, and community. Social support is a crucial factor in resilience.

Empowerment

Engage in activities that promote a sense of empowerment and control, such as volunteering, advocacy, and pursuing personal goals.

RECOVERY STRATEGIES

Journaling

Writing about your thoughts and feelings can help process emotions and gain insights into your experiences.

Creative Outlets

Engage in creative activities such as art, music, or dance to express emotions and promote healing.

Physical Activity

Regular physical activity can reduce stress, improve mood, and enhance overall well-being. Activities like yoga, tai chi, and walking can be particularly beneficial.

Healthy Coping Mechanisms

Avoid unhealthy behaviours such as substance abuse, overeating, and isolation. Focus instead on developing healthy coping mechanisms to manage stress and emotions.

Creating a Support System

As discussed in Chapter 8, identify trusted individuals who can provide emotional support, practical assistance, and encouragement.

Community Resources

Utilize community networks and resources such as crisis centres, hotlines, and support groups to access additional support.

Safety Plan

Develop a safety plan that includes steps to take in case of a crisis, contact information for emergency services, and a list of supportive individuals to reach out to.

———

I want to remind you that trauma, in any form, can have profound and lasting effects. It doesn't matter if the incident was something seemingly minor, like an unsettling interaction during a morning run, or something more significant that rocked your entire world. Each person's trauma is real, and it matters.

As evidenced by my friend – who experienced a routine jog that turned into an experience that silently unravelled her peace of mind – one disturbing encounter with a stranger in a passing car didn't just interrupt her run, it slowly chipped away at her sense of safety and security, both in her daily life and in herself. What felt like a small moment of fear crept into unexpected parts of her world, altering her habits, relationships, and even her confidence.

This is what trauma does. It doesn't always announce itself loudly or right away. It can simmer beneath the surface, reshaping how we see the world, how we trust, and how we live. Trauma is personal, and it doesn't have to look like anyone else's to be valid.

I like to think of healing from trauma like tending to a garden that has been hit by a storm. The flowers may seem battered and bent, and at first glance, you may wonder if they'll bloom again. But with time, nurturing, and care, the garden can regrow − sometimes stronger and more resilient than before. The roots are still there, capable of thriving, just as you are.

The journey to coping with trauma isn't always straightforward, but it is absolutely possible to heal, to grow, and to regain the control that trauma can take from us. Recognizing what you're experiencing is the first step. Seeking help, whether through counselling, community support, or building personal resilience, is how you begin the process of recovery.

Remember this: healing is a process, not a destination. It's okay to take small steps, and it's okay to lean on others for help along the way. Most importantly, don't underestimate the power of your own strength and resilience. Just like my friend, whose simple morning run turned into a long-term struggle for peace, you, too, can find your way back to a place of empowerment and safety, one step at a time.

CONCLUSION

In a world where safety concerns for women are multifaceted and ever-present, equipping ourselves with knowledge and practical strategies is crucial for navigating life's challenges. This book has aimed to provide you with a comprehensive guide to women's safety, covering a wide range of topics from self-defence techniques and cybersecurity to coping with trauma and building a support network. In reading these ten chapters, I hope I empowered you to take charge of your safety and well-being, build resilience, confidence, and independence.

Ultimately, the key to women's safety lies in empowerment. Taking control of our environment, assessing risks, and encouraging independence and vigilance are vital steps in creating a secure and fulfilling life. By empowering ourselves and others with knowledge, skills, and support, we can foster a culture of safety and resilience.

As you close this book, remember that safety is an ongoing journey, not a destination. Continue to educate yourself, practice the techniques learned, and stay connected with your support network. By doing so, you can navigate the world with greater confidence, resilience, and empowerment. Your safety is a priority, and taking proactive steps today will ensure a brighter, safer tomorrow.

Nichelle Laus

ABOUT THE AUTHOR

Nichelle Laus is a former police officer turned women's fitness coach, safety advocate, and entrepreneur. With a background in law enforcement and kickboxing, Nichelle draws from personal experiences of overcoming childhood trauma to empower women through health, fitness, and personal safety. She co-owns 416 Tactical with her husband, sharing practical safety tips on social media while inspiring confidence in women everywhere. Nichelle's journey has led her to help thousands of women become their best selves, building strength both mentally and physically.

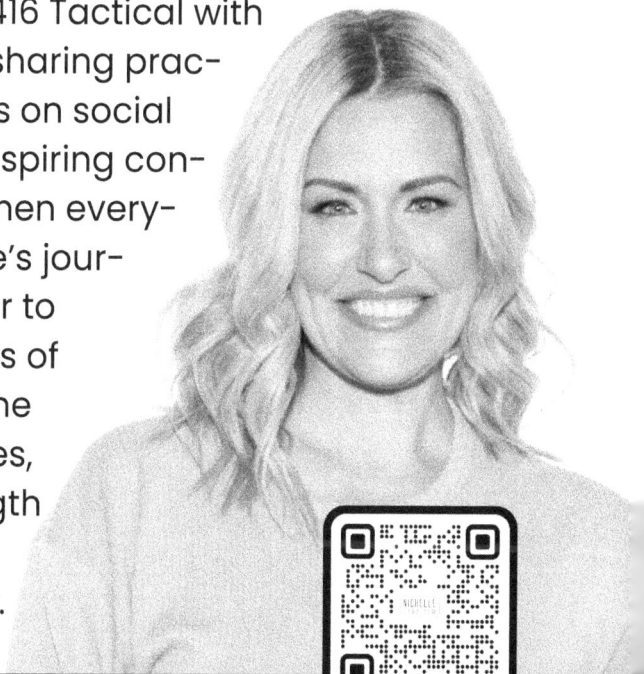

RESOURCES

Your safety and well-being are always a priority, and I understand that the journey to feeling empowered and secure can be a deeply personal one. While the strategies and techniques in this book can serve as a foundation, I want you to have access to a wider network of support whenever you need it. Whether you're seeking guidance, additional training, or immediate assistance, the following resources are here to provide you with the strength, knowledge, and help you deserve. Remember, you are never alone on this path, and there is always someone ready to support you.

Websites and Hotlines

Common Sense Self-Defense (CSSD)
nichellelaus.com/safety/

Canadian Women's Foundation (Canada)
canadianwomen.org

National Domestic Violence Hotline (USA)
thehotline.org
1-800-799-7233 (SAFE)

*RAINN (Rape, Abuse & Incest National Network)
(USA)*
rainn.org
1-800-656-HOPE (4673)

Love Is Respect (USA)
loveisrespect.org
Hotline: 1-866-331-9474

Victim Support (UK)
victimsupport.org.uk
08 08 16 89 111

Women's Aid (UK)
womensaid.org.uk

White Ribbon Campaign (Global)
whiteribbon.ca

UN Women – Ending Violence Against Women (Global)
unwomen.org

WAVE Network (Women Against Violence Europe)
wave-network.org

Books

The Gift of Fear by Gavin de Becker
Boundaries: When to Say Yes, How to Say No to Take Control of Your Life by Dr. Henry Cloud and Dr. John Townsend
Self-Defense for Women: Fight Back by Willy Cahill
No More Workbooks: How to Stand Up for Yourself & Set Boundaries by Brigid Dineen
Strong on Defense by Sanford Strong

Nonprofit Organizations

Safe Horizon (USA)
safehorizon.org

Women for Women International (Global)
womenforwomen.org

Futures Without Violence (USA)
futureswithoutviolence.org

Hollaback! (Global)
ihollaback.org

Apps

Circle of 6 (Global)
A safety app that lets users alert friends when in danger, send pre-programmed emergency texts, and track their location.

Noonlight (USA)
A personal safety app that connects users to emergency services by just pressing a button.

bSafe (Global)
Includes GPS tracking, emergency alerts, and voice-activated SOS alarms to enhance personal safety.

REFERENCES

1
Canadian Women's Foundation. "The Facts about Gender-Based Violence." Canadian Women's Foundation, 4 Jan. 2024, canadianwomen.org/the-facts/gender-based-violence/#:~:text=Women%20self%2Dreport%20violent%20victimization,higher%20for%20women%20than%20men. Accessed 7 May 2024.

2
Briggs Myers, Isabel, Mary H. McCaulley, Naomi L. Quenk, and Allen L. Hammer. MBTI® Manual: A Guide to the Development and Use of the Myers-Briggs Type Indicator Instrument. 3rd ed. Palo Alto, CA: Consulting Psychologists Press, 1998.

3
Wiggins, Jerry S., ed. The Five-Factor Model of Personality: Theoretical Perspectives. New York: Guilford Press, 1996.

4
Buckingham, Marcus, and Donald O. Clifton. Now, Discover Your Strengths. New York: Free Press, 2001.

5
"In a Nutshell: Strengths-Based Thinking." Human Performance Technology by DTS, 26 May 2014, blog.hptbydts.com/in-a-nutshell-strengths-based-thinking-strengths-movement. Accessed 27 May 2024.

6
Girls. Season 3, Episode 6, "Free Snacks." Directed by Richard Shepard. Written by Lena Dunham. Aired on February 9, 2014, on HBO.

leadher

PUBLISHING

Published in partnership with *LeadHer Publishing*, an boutique publishing agency dedicated to helping badass women writers share their voices.

To find out more, visit leadherpublishing.com.

www.ingramcontent.com/pod-product-compliance
Lightning Source LLC
Chambersburg PA
CBHW060232030426
42335CB00014B/1416